Selected Tables and Figures from

The Practice of Emergency and Critical Care Neurology

T0177553

Selected Tables and Figures from

The Practice of Emergency and Critical Care Neurology

Second Edition

Eelco F. M. Wijdicks, MD, PhD, FACP, FNCS, FANA

Professor of Neurology, Mayo Clinic College
 of Medicine
Chair, Division of Critical Care Neurology
Consultant, Neurosciences Intensive Care Unit
Mayo Clinic Hospital, Saint Marys Campus
Mayo Clinic Rochester, Minnesota

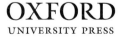

OXFORD
UNIVERSITY PRESS

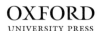

OXFORD
UNIVERSITY PRESS

Oxford University Press is a department of the University of Oxford. It furthers
the University's objective of excellence in research, scholarship, and education
by publishing worldwide. Oxford is a registered trade mark of Oxford University
Press in the UK and certain other countries.

Published in the United States of America by Oxford University Press
198 Madison Avenue, New York, NY 10016, United States of America.

© 2016 Mayo Foundation for Medical Education and Research

First Edition published in 2010

Library of Congress Cataloging-in-Publication Data
Wijdicks, Eelco F. M., 1954– , author
Selected tables and figures from The practice of emergency and critical care
neurology / Eelco F. M. Wijdicks.—Second edition.
p. ; cm.
ISBN 978–0–19–060208–6 (alk. paper)
I. Wijdicks, Eelco F. M., 1954– Practice of emergency and critical care
neurology. Supplement to (work):   II. Title.
[DNLM: 1. Neurologic Manifestations—Tables.   2. Central Nervous System
Diseases—diagnosis—Tables.   3. Central Nervous System
Diseases—therapy—Tables.   4. Critical Care—methods—Tables.
5. Emergency Treatment—methods—Tables. WL 16]
RC350.N49
616.8'0428—dc23
2015036949

9 8 7 6 5 4 3 2 1

Printed by Sheridan, USA

Preface

This pocketbook includes a selection of tables and figures from

THE PRACTICE OF EMERGENCY AND CRITICAL CARE NEUROLOGY, SECOND EDITION

There continues to be a need to have information immediately available—put together in a book functionally designed to fit in a pocket or to download on a mobile device allowing easy scroll through. Such is self-evident but a quick reference is not easy to find on line or may even be unreliable and outdated. Therefore this new edition will continue to provide a pocket size edition—on hard copy and digitally.

This book is a selection of tables and figures taken from the larger textbook (*The practice of emergency and critical care neurology second edition*). This pocket book is of course not a substitute for study of the larger text and thus the material herein cannot be fully appreciated without prior reading of this textbook.

The pocket book compiles the main conclusions of the chapters and includes the most practically useful tables and figures to quickly look things up, verify a dose, write an order set and to provide emergency care of critically ill neurologic patients. Important formulas are included as well as commonly used rating scales. The booklet has blank pages to allow the practitioner to take a few notes.

I hope this booklet serves a purpose.

Contents

Contents

Part III Evaluation of Presenting Symptoms Indicating Critical Emergency

Part V General Principles of Management of Critically Ill Neurologic Patients in the Neurosciences Intensive Care Unit

Part VI Technologies in the Neurosciences Intensive Care Unit

Part X Critical Care Support

Part XI Management of Systemic Complications

Part XII Decisions at the End of Life and Other Responsibilities

PART XIII Formulas and Scales

Chapter 1

The Presenting Neurologic Emergency

PRACTICAL NOTES

- Neurologic symptoms often fluctuate, and an improvement in symptoms may not necessarily mean the patient is improving.
- Signs and symptoms indicating an neurologic emergency are worsening or changing neurologic signs, any abnormal level of consciousness, acute split second onset headache, acute vertigo, acute cranial nerve deficit and an inability to stand or walk.

CAPSULE 1.1   INJURY SEVERITY SCORE

Region	Injury Description	AIS
Head and neck	Cerebral contusion	4
Face	No injury	0
Chest	Flail chest	4
Abdomen	Minor contusion of liver	2
	Complex ruptured spleen	5
Extremity	Fractured femur	3
External	No injury	0

Rating for the Abbreviated Injury Scale (AIS)

AIS Score	Injury
1	Minor
2	Moderate
3	Serious
4	Severe
5	Critical
6	Unsurvivable

To obtain an injury severity score, square the 3 highest scores and add them. In this example $25 + 16 + 16 = 57$

TABLE 1.2. SIGNS AND SYMPTOMS THAT MAY CONSTITUTE A NEUROLOGIC EMERGENCY

Worsening and changing neurologic signs
Acutely dilated pupil or anisocoria
Acute eye movement abnormality
Abnormal level of consciousness
Seizure
Severe, unexpected, split-second headache
Acute vertigo
Acute cranial nerve deficit
Inability to stand or walk

TABLE 1.3. ERRORS THAT MAY OCCUR IN THE EMERGENCY DEPARTMENT

Failure to recognize acute brain injury on computed tomographic scanning
Failure to perform a cerebrospinal fluid examination
Failure to recognize acute hydrocephalus
Failure to recognize locked-in syndrome
Failure to recognize brainstem involvement
Failure to recognize status epilepticus
Failure to recognize spinal cord compression
Failure to recognize neurointerventional options
Failure to recognize brain death and potential for organ donation

Chapter 2

Criteria of Triage Emergency

PRACTICAL NOTES

- Triage to the NICU should be based on certain criteria. Any patient with a neurologic disorder and unstable vital signs (pulse rate, blood pressure, respiratory rate, core temperature) or a progressive neurologic presentation should be admitted.
- Communication between the physician in the emergency department and NICU attending physician requires special effort.
- Triage out the NICU requires assessment of neurologic and respiratory stability and absence of IV antihypertensives or IV cardiac drugs.

TABLE 2.1. COMMON REASONS FOR ADMISSION TO THE NEUROSCIENCES INTENSIVE CARE UNIT

Aneurysmal subarachnoid hemorrhage
Drowsiness, stupor, or coma
Mechanical ventilation
Any neurologic deterioration
Seizures
Neurogenic pulmonary edema
Aspiration pneumonia
Cardiac arrhythmias
Abnormal electrocardiogram
S/P coil placement
S/P clipping of aneurysm

Ganglionic or lobar hemorrhage
Drowsiness, stupor, or coma
Mechanical ventilation
CT scan evidence of brain shift
Hypertensive surges

Acute bacterial meningitis
Drowsiness, stupor, or coma
Mechanical ventilation
CT scan evidence of edema
Any neurologic deterioration despite antibiotic
    therapy
Seizures
Shock
Pulmonary infiltrates

Brain abscess
Drowsiness, stupor, or coma
Mechanical ventilation
CT scan evidence of mass effect
Seizures
S/P drainage
S/P stereotactic puncture

(continued)

TABLE 2.1. (CONTINUED)

Recurrent seizures

Coagulopathy or warfarin use

S/P ventriculostomy

S/P craniotomy

Cerebellum or brainstem hemorrhage

Drowsiness, stupor, or coma

Mechanical ventilation

CT or clinical signs of brainstem compression

Cardiac arrhythmia

S/P ventriculostomy

S/P craniotomy

Major hemispheric ischemic stroke syndromes

Drowsiness, stupor, or coma

Mechanical ventilation

CT scan evidence of early swelling
or hemorrhagic conversion

Seizures

Acute encephalitis

Drowsiness, stupor, or coma

Mechanical ventilation

CT scan evidence of swelling

Seizures

S/P brain biopsy

Acute spinal cord disorders

Mechanical ventilation

Cervical lesion

Ascending paralysis

Associated traumatic brain injury

Pulmonary infiltrates

Dysautonomia or acute bladder distension

Anticipated surgical intervention

Acute white matter disorders

Drowsiness, stupor, or coma

Mechanical ventilation

Cardiac failure or arrhythmias
S/P craniotomy
S/P endovascular intervention

Basilar artery occlusion
Drowsiness, stupor, or coma
Mechanical ventilation
S/P thrombolysis
S/P endovascular intervention

Cerebellar infarct
Drowsiness, stupor, or coma
Mechanical ventilation
CT scan or clinical evidence
of brainstem compression
Cardiac arrhythmias
S/P ventriculostomy
S/P craniotomy

Seizures
Need to monitor plasma exchange

Acute obstructive hydrocephalus
Drowsiness, stupor, or coma
Mechanical ventilation
Ventriculostomy

Malignant brain tumors
Drowsiness, stupor, or coma
Mechanical ventilation
CT scan evidence of cerebral edema
Recurrent seizures

Status epilepticus
Drowsiness, stupor, or coma
Mechanical ventilation
Need for more intravenous antiepileptic drugs
Need for video/EEG monitoring

(continued)

TABLE 2.1 (CONTINUED)

Cerebral venous thrombosis

Drowsiness, stupor, or coma

Mechanical ventilation

CT scan evidence of hemorrhagic infarct

Seizures

Suspected pulmonary embolus

S/P endovascular intervention

Guillain-Barré syndrome

VC < 20 mL/kg, $PI_{max} < -30$ cm H_2O, $PE_{max} < 40$ cm
H_2O or 30% decrease in any of these values

Mechanical ventilation

Pulmonary infiltrates

Rapid clinical progression

Dysautonomia

Pneumonia or sepsis

Traumatic brain injury

Drowsiness, stupor, or coma

Mechanical ventilation

CT scan evidence of contusions or early brain swelling

Seizures

Evidence of multitrauma

S/P craniotomy

Myasthenia gravis

Myasthenic crisis with neuromuscular respiratory
failure (VC< 20 mL/kg or 30% decrease)

Bulbar weakness

Mechanical ventilation

CT, computed tomography; EEG, electroencephalography; ICH, intracranial hemorrhage; PE_{max}, maximal expiratory pressure;
PI_{max}, maximal inspiratory pressure; S/P, status post; VC, vital capacity.

TABLE 2.2. CONSIDERATIONS
FOR TRANSFER OF THE NEUROLOGIC
PATIENT (ESSENTIALS OF PATIENT
HANDOFFS)

Detailed neurologic examination and clinical course

FOUR score (EMBR 0–16)*

Mechanical ventilator settings

Review of dose of vasopressors

Review of recent use of neuromusculzar blocking
   agents and sedatives

Review of antiepileptic drugs

Review of neuroimaging

Consult with interventional neuroradiologist

Meeting with family members for their
   understanding of patient's condition and
   assessment of level of care.

*For FOUR score description, see Chapter 12.

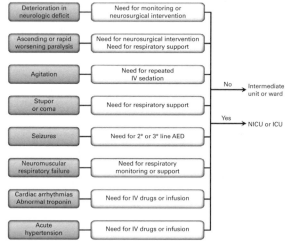

Figure 2.1: Common signs and symptoms associated with acute neurologic illness when triaging patients to an intensive care unit or other wards.

AED, antiepileptic drug; ICU, intensive care unit; IV, intravenous; NICU, neurosciences intensive care unit.

Part II Evaluation of Presenting Symptoms Indicating Urgency

Chapter 3

Confused and Febrile

PRACTICAL NOTES

- Most confused and febrile patients have an underlying systemic infection.
- Confusion may indicate a more specific language disorder.
- Multisystem involvement and confusion may indicate certain infectious agents.
- Abnormal immune status should be investigated because its presence has a different set of diagnostic possibilities.

TABLE 3.1. OBSERVATIONS AND CLUES IN THE CONFUSED FEBRILE PATIENT

Debilitated, wasted, underfed (drug abuse, alcoholism, cancer)

Exposure to ticks, mosquitoes and beginning of endemic encephalitis (arboviruses)

Exposure to wilderness, tropics, animal bite (rabies)

Exposure to excessive heat (heat stroke)

Recent travel or immigration from developing country (neurocysticercosis, fungal meningitis)

Recent vaccination (ADEM)

Prior transplantation or AIDS (*Toxoplasma* encephalitis or *Aspergillus*)

ADEM, acute disseminated encephalomyelitis; AIDS, acquired immunodeficiency syndrome.

TABLE 3.2. SYSTEMIC ILLNESSES WITH FEVER AND CONFUSION

Septic shock
Lobar pneumonia
Acute osteomyelitis
Abdominal suppuration
Endocarditis
Erysipelas
Measles
Psittacosis
Influenza
Yellow fever
Typhoid fever
Cholera
Heat stroke
Thyrotoxicosis

TABLE 3.3. GENERAL CLINICAL SIGNS
INDICATING CAUSES IN CONFUSED
FEBRILE PATIENTS

Signs	Disorder
Skin rash	Rickettsial diseases
	Vasculitis
	Aspergillosis
Petechiae	Thrombocytopenic purpura
	Meningococcemia
	Endocarditis
	Drug eruption from intoxication
	Leukemia
Splenomegaly	Toxoplasmosis
	Tuberculosis
	Sepsis
	Human immunodeficiency virus infection
	Lymphoma
Pulmonary infiltrates	*Legionella* species
	Fungi
	Tuberculosis
	Mycoplasma
	Pneumonia
	Q fever
	Tick-borne diseases

TABLE 3.4. DIAGNOSTIC EVALUATION TO CONSIDER IN DETERMINING THE MICROBIAL ETIOLOGY IN PATIENTS WITH ENCEPHALITIS

Class of Microorganism	General Diagnostic Evaluation
Viruses	Culture of respiratory secretions and nasopharynx, throat, and stool specimens[a]
	DFA of sputum for respiratory viruses
	PCR of respiratory specimens
	Culture and/or DFA of skin lesions (if present) for herpes simplex virus and varicella-zoster virus
	Serologic testing for HIV[b]
	Serologic testing for Epstein-Barr virus
	Serologic testing (acute and convalescent phase) for St. Louis encephalitis virus,[c] Eastern equine encephalitis virus,[c]
	Venezuelan equine encephalitis virus,[c] La Crosse virus,[c]
	West Nile virus[c]
	CSF IgM for West Nile virus,[c] St. Louis encephalitis virus,[c] varicella-zoster virus
	CSF PCR for herpes simplex virus 1, herpes simplex virus 2, varicella-zoster virus, Epstein-Barr virus,[d] enteroviruses
Bacteria	Blood cultures
	CSF cultures

	Serologic testing (acute and convalescent phase) for *Mycoplasma pneumoniae*
	PCR of respiratory secretions for *Mycoplasma pneumoniae*
Rickettsiae and ehrlichiae[c]	Serologic testing (acute and convalescent phase) for *Rickettsia rickettsi, Ehrlichia chaffeensis*, and *Anaplasma phagocytophilum*
	DFA and PCR of skin biopsy specimen (if rash present) for *Rickettsia rickettsiae*
	Blood smears for morulae
	PCR of whole blood and CSF specimens for *Ehrlichia* and *Anaplasma* species[e]
Spirochetes	Serum RPR and FTA-ABS
	Serologic testing for *Borrelia burgdorferi* (ELISA and Western blot)
	CSF VDRL
	CSF *Borrelia burgdorferi* serologic testing (ELISA and Western blot); IgG antibody index
	CSF FTA-ABS[f]
Mycobacteria	Chest radiograph
	PCR and culture of respiratory secretions
	CSF AFB smear and culture
	CSF PCR (Gen-Probe Amplified *Mycobacterium tuberculosis* Direct Test)
Fungi	Blood cultures
	CSF cultures
	Serum and CSF cryptococcal antigen
	Urine and CSF *Histoplasma* antigen[g]

TABLE 3.4. (CONTINUED)

	Serum and CSF complement fixing or immunodiffusion antibodies for *Coccidioides* species
Protozoa	Serum IgG for *Toxoplasma gondii*[h]

Note: These tests may not be required in all patients with encephalitis; certain tests should not be performed unless a consistent epidemiology is present. Additional tests should be considered on the basis of epidemiology, risk factors, clinical features, general diagnostic studies, neuroimaging features, and CSF analysis. Recommended tests should not supplant clinical judgment; not all tests are recommended in all age groups. AFB, acid-fast bacilli; CSF, cerebrospinal fluid; DFA, direct fluorescent antibody; ELISA, enzyme-linked immunosorbent assay; FTA-ABS, fluorescent treponemal antibody, absorbed; PCR, polymerase chain reaction; RPR, rapid plasma reagin; VDRL, Venereal Disease Research Laboratory.

[a] Additional diagnostic studies for immunocompromised patients are CSF PCR for cytomegalovirus JC virus, human herpesvirus 6, and West Nile virus.

[b] In patients who are HIV seronegative but in whom there is a high index of suspicion for HIV infection, plasma HIV RNA testing should be performed.

[c] Depending on time of year or geographic locale.

[d] Results should be interpreted in conjunction with Epstein-Barr virus serologic testing; quantitative PCR should be done, because a low CSF copy number may be an incidental finding.

[e] Low yield of CSF PCR.

[f] CSF FTA-ABS is sensitive but not specific for the diagnosis of neurosyphilis; a nonreactive CSF test result may exclude the diagnosis, but a reactive test result does not establish the diagnosis.

[g] Depends on a history of residence in or travel to an area of endemicity.

[h] Positive results may suggest the possibility of reactivation disease in an immunocompromised host.

Adapted from Tunkel et al. The management of encephalitis: clinical practice guidelines by the Infectious Diseases Society of America. *Clin Infect Dis* 2008:47:303–327, with permission of publisher.

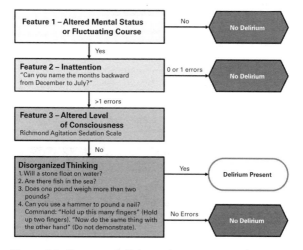

Figure 3.1: Two-step delirium triage screen used in emergency departments.

From Han et al. (2103) with permission.

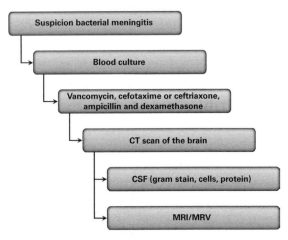

Figure 3.2: Critical steps in the evaluation of the febrile confused patient suspicious of acute bacterial meningitis.

CSF, cerebrospinal fluid; CT, computed tomography; MRI, magnetic resonance imaging; MRV, magnetic resonance venography.

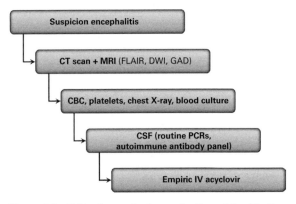

Figure 3.3: Critical steps in the evaluation of the febrile confused patient suspicious of encephalitis.

CBC, complete blood count; CSF, cerebrospinal fluid; CT, computed tomography; DWI, diffusion-weighted imaging; FLAIR, fluid-attenuated inversion recovery; GAD, gadolinium enhancement; PCR, polymerase chain reaction.

Chapter 4

A Terrible Headache

PRACTICAL NOTES

- The evaluation of severe headaches in the ED is common and often not due to a major neurologic illness. The challenge is to identify that single patient with an emergency.
- The distinctive nature of a "thunderclap headache" needs to be recognized.
- Acute headache syndromes may be refractory migraine or cluster headache and good treatment options exist in the ED.
- Acute severe headache may have a non-neurologic cause.

TABLE 4.1. WARNING SIGNS IN ACUTE HEADACHE

Signs and Symptoms	Diagnosis to Consider
Split-second onset, unexpected, and excruciating	Aneurysmal subarachnoid hemorrhage
Loss of consciousness, vertigo, or vomiting	Cerebellar hematoma
Acute cranial nerve deficit (particularly oculomotor palsy)	Carotid artery aneurysm
Carotid bruit (in young individuals)	Carotid artery dissection
Fever and skin rash	Meningitis
Shock, Addison's disease	Pituitary apoplexy
Fall and coagulopathy or anticoagulation	Subdural, epidural, or intracerebral hematoma
Facial edema and vesicular rash	Herpes zoster ophthalmicus

TABLE 4.2. ACUTE SEVERE HEADACHE SYNDROMES
FROM NON-NEUROLOGIC CAUSES

Disorder	Location	Time Profile	Characteristic Features
Acute-angle glaucoma	Eye, frontal	Acute	Red eye, midrange pupil, decreased vision
Temporal arteritis	Temporal, frontal	Rapidly built up	Temporal artery painful, sedimentation rate > 55 mm/hr
Acute sinusitis	Frontal and maxilla	Hours	Fever, pressure pain on maxillary or frontal sinus
Pheochromocytoma	Entire head	Rapidly increasing intensity	Sweating, pallor, systolic blood pressure > 200 mm Hg

TABLE 4.3. SYMPTOMATIC THUNDERCLAP HEADACHE OTHER THAN ANEURYSMAL SUBARACHNOID HEMORRHAGE

Diagnosis	Clues in History	Clues in Examination	MR Features
PRES	Poorly controlled hypertension	Systolic blood pressure > 200 mm Hg	Abnormalities predominantly in parieto-occipital lobes
Cerebral vasoconstriction syndrome	Recurrence	Use of vasoactive agents, migraine	Convexity subarachnoid hemorrhage, cerebral hematoma or infarct
Cerebral venous thrombosis	None	Increased CSF opening pressure	Transverse or sagittal sinus obstruction on MRV
Retroclival hematoma	None	CSF xanthochromia	Clot posteriorly and at level of clivus

Pituitary apoplexy	Cranial nerve deficit	Hypotension, hyponatremia	Pituitary tumor with hemorrhage
CSF hypotension	Marfan characteristics	Headache posture-related	Meningeal enhancement; subdural hematomas "sagging brain"
Carotid or vertebral artery dissection	Trauma, chiropractic therapy	Horner's syndrome, carotid bruit, dysarthria	Recent cerebral infarcts; double lumen sign on MRI

CSF, cerebrospinal fluid; MRI, magnetic resonance imaging; MRV, magnetic resonance venography; PRES, posterior reversible encephalopathy syndrome.

TABLE 4.4. "BENIGN" ACUTE HEADACHE SYNDROMES

Disorder	Location	Time Profile	Quality	Characteristic Features
Cluster headache	Oculofrontal, temporal	30–90 minutes	Severe, stabbing	Rocking, restless, Horner syndrome, rhinorrhea
Chronic paroxysmal hemicrania	Unilateral	2–30 minutes	Severe	Conjunctival injection, not restless, lacrimation on symptomatic side (common in females)
Acute migraine	Mostly unilateral	6–30 hours	Moderately severe	Nausea and photophobia in 80%
Trigeminal neuralgia	Face	Seconds	Severe, electrical	Provoked by chewing, cold wind against face, shaving, tooth brushing

TABLE 4.5. REASONS FOR FAILURE
TO RECOGNIZE SUBARACHNOID
HEMORRHAGE ON COMPUTED
TOMOGRAPHY SCANS

Blood in prepontine cistern is not visualized but is
present on repeat CT scan

Blood in a part of the pentagon is not visualized from
tilting of the gantry but is present on repeat CT
scan

Absent unilateral sylvian fissure from isodense SAH

Sedimentation of blood in dependent part of the
posterior ventricular horns

Blood in basal cisterns misinterpreted as contrast
enhancement

Blood on tentorium misinterpreted as calcification

CT, computed tomography; SAH, subarachnoid hemorrhage.

TABLE 4.6. ABORTIVE THERAPIES IN UNRELENTING HEAD PAIN

Disorder	Therapy Options
Migraine	Sumatriptan (6 mg SC) or nasal spray 5 mg; repeat after 1 hour, if needed
	Droperidol (2.75–8.25 mg IM)
	Meperidine (100 mg IM) and hydroxyzine (50 mg IM)
	Valproate sodium (1,000 mg IV in 50 mL normal saline over 60 min)
	Dihydroergotamine (1–3 mg IV at hourly intervals) and metoclopramide (10 mg IM)
	Butorphanol nasal spray 1mg
	Ketorolac 30–60 mg IM
	Prochlorperazine 10 mg (in 10 mL saline infused in 2 min)
Cluster headache	Oxygen therapy (7 L/min face mask)
	Metoclopramide (10 mg IM)
	Sumatriptan (6 mg SC)

	Nasal butorphanol (1 mg/1 puff)
	Intranasal lidocaine 4% (4 sprays)
Trigeminal neuralgia	Fosphenytoin IV loading (15–20 mg/kg IV)
	Carbamazepine (1,200 mg/day)
	Lamotrigine (50–100 mg/day)
	Topiramate (50–100 mg/day)
Acute herpetic neuralgia	Tramadol (50–400 mg/day)
	Pregabalin (75–600 mg/day)
	Gabapentin (300–3600 mg/day)

IM, intramuscular; IV, intravenous; SC, subcutaneous.
References[39,54]

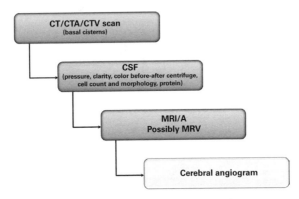

Figure 4.2: Critical steps in the evaluation of severe new acute headache.

CSF, cerebrospinal fluid; CT, computed tomography; MRI/A, magnetic resonance imaging/angiography; MRV, magnetic resonance venography.

Chapter 5

Blacked Out and Slumped Down

PRACTICAL NOTES

- Cardiac arrhythmias can mimic seizures or caused by seizures
- Patients with ictal bradycardia likely need a pacemaker.
- Syncope rarely heralds an acute neurologic disease but may be part of an undiagnosed chronic neurologic illness.

TABLE 5.1. CAUSES OF SYNCOPE

Neurally Mediated (Reflex) Syncope

Vasovagal syncope (common faint)

Carotid sinus syncope

Situational syncope

– Cough, sneeze, swallow, defecation, visceral pain

– Micturition

– After exercise

– After a meal

– Other causes

Glossopharyngeal neuralgia

(continued)

TABLE 5.1. (CONTINUED)

Orthostatic Hypotension

Autonomic failure
– Primary autonomic failure syndromes (e.g., pure
  autonomic failure, multiple-system atrophy,
  Parkinson's disease with autonomic failure)
– Secondary autonomic failure syndromes (e.g.,
  diabetic neuropathy, amyloid neuropathy)
– Drugs and alcohol
– After exercise
– After a meal
Volume depletion
– Hemorrhage, diarrhea, Addison disease

Cardiac Arrhythmias

Sinus node dysfunction (including bradycardia-
  tachycardia syndrome)
Atrioventricular conduction system disease
Paroxysmal supraventricular and ventricular
  tachycardias
Congenital syndromes (e.g., long QT syndrome)
Malfunction of an implanted device (e.g., pacemaker,
  implantable cardioverter-defibrillator)
Drug-induced arrhythmias

(*continued*)

TABLE 5.1. (CONTINUED)

Structural Cardiac or Cardiopulmonary Disease

Obstructive cardiac valvular disease
Acute myocardial infarction
Obstructive cardiomyopathy
Atrial myxoma
Acute aortic dissection
Pericardial disease
Pulmonary embolus and pulmonary hypertension

Data from Soteriades ES, Evans JC, Larson MG, et al. Incidence and prognosis of syncope. *N Engl J Med* 2002;347:878–885; and Strickberger SA, Benson W, Biaggioni I, et al. American Heart Association Councils on Clinical Cardiology, Cardiovascular Nursing, Cardiovascular Disease in the young, and, Stroke; Quality of Care and Outcomes Research Interdisciplinary Working Group; American College of Cardiology Foundation in collaboration with the Heart Rhythm Society; American Autonomic Society. AHA/ACCF scientific statement on the evaluation of syncope. *Circulation* 2006; 113:316–327. With permission of the publishers.

TABLE 5.2. ELECTROCARDIOGRAM ABNORMALITIES SUGGESTIVE OF ARRHYTHMIC SYNCOPE

Bifascicular block (defined as either a left bundle-branch block or a right bundle-branch block combined with a left anterior or left posterior fascicular block)

Other intraventricular conduction abnormalities (e.g., a QRS duration ≥ 0.12 seconds)

Mobitz I second-degree atrioventricular block

Asymptomatic sinus bradycardia (< 50 beats/min), sinoatrial block, or sinus pause (≥ 3 seconds) in the absence of negatively chronotropic medications

Pre-excited QRS complexes

Prolonged QT interval

Right bundle-branch block pattern with ST elevation in leads V1–V3 (Brugada syndrome)

Negative T waves in right precordial leads, epsilon waves and ventricular late potentials suggestive of arrhythmogenic right ventricular dysplasia

Q waves suggestive of myocardial infarction

Data from Soteriades ES, Evans JC, Larson MG, et al. Incidence and prognosis of syncope. *N Engl J Med* 2002;347:878–885; and Strickberger SA, Benson W, Biaggioni I, et al. American Heart Association Councils on Clinical Cardiology, Cardiovascular Nursing, Cardiovascular Disease in the young, and, Stroke; Quality of Care and Outcomes Research Interdisciplinary Working Group; American College of Cardiology Foundation in collaboration with the Heart Rhythm Society; American Autonomic Society. AHA/ACCF scientific statement on the evaluation of syncope. *Circulation* 2006; 113:316–327. With permission of the publishers.

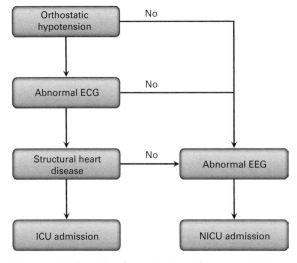

Figure 5.3: Algorithm for evaluation of syncope in the emergency department.

ECG, electrocardiogram; EEG, electroencephalogram; ICU, intensive care unit; NICU, neurosciences intensive care unit.

Chapter 6

See Nothing, See Double, See Shapes

PRACTICAL NOTES

- Neurologic causes of acute monocular (optic neuropathy) or binocular (occipital lobes) vision loss are less common than ophthalmologic causes.
- Painful ophthalmoplegia has a broad spectrum of causes and needs urgent evaluation.
- Positive visual phenomena rarely indicate acute neurologic disease and more often are associated with neurotoxicity.

CAPSULE 6.1	DEGREE OF VISUAL LOSS
20/200	Legal blindness
20/800	Finger counting
2/1000	Arm movements
20/∞	Light perception
0	No light perception

TABLE 6.1. OPHTHALMOLOGIC DISORDERS

Diagnosis	Findings
Central retinal artery occlusion	Afferent pupil defect
	Retinal edema
	Optic disk pallor and cherry-red spots
Retinal vein occlusion	"Blood-and-thunder" fundus (extensive intraretinal hemorrhages)
Retinal detachment	Translucent gray wrinkled retina
Ischemic optic neuropathy	Pale optic nerve
	Milky, swelling
	Scalp tenderness and absent temporal artery pulsation (giant cell arteritis)
Optic neuritis	Normal findings ("patient sees nothing, doctor sees nothing")
	Early pallor
Vitreous hemorrhage	Diabetes, hypertension

TABLE 6.2. DIPLOPIA DUE TO CRANIAL NERVE PALSY

Cranial Nerve	Position of Eye	Diplopia	Additional Features
III	Down and out	Crossed	Ptosis, dilated fixed pupil
IV	Higher	Vertical	Head tilted away from affected side, chin down
VI	Inward	Uncrossed*	Head turned to affected side

* The image appears on the same side as the eye that sees it.

TABLE 6.3. URGENT DISORDERS IN ACUTE DIPLOPIA

Acute third-nerve palsy	Basilar artery aneurysm, posterior communicating artery aneurysm*
	Pituitary apoplexy
	Acute midbrain infarct or hemorrhage
	Mucormycosis*
	Carotid cavernous fistula
	Granulomatous inflammation (Tolosa-Hunt)
	Diabetic microvascular disease†
Acute fourth-nerve palsy	Trauma
	Meningitis, infectious or neoplastic*
	Herpes zoster ophthalmicus*
Acute sixth-nerve palsy	Carotid aneurysm
	Cavernous sinus thrombosis*
	Nasopharyngeal carcinoma
	Increased intracranial pressure

*Also known as the painful ophthalmoplegias.[11]
†More often pupil-sparing.

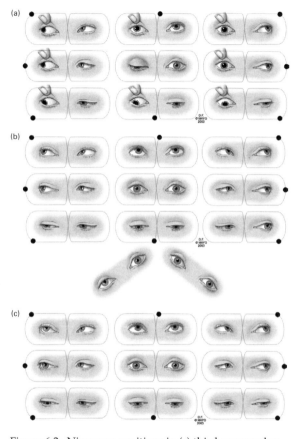

Figure 6.2: Nine gaze positions in (a) third-nerve palsy, (b) fourth-nerve palsy, and (c) sixth-nerve palsy (patient follows black dot).

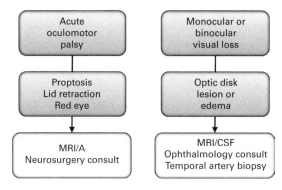

Figure 6.7. Critical steps in acute neuro-ophthalmology.

CSF, cerebrospinal fluid; MRI/A, magnetic resonance imaging/angiography.

Chapter 7

Spinning

PRACTICAL NOTES

- The type and direction of a newly discovered nystagmus provides clues to the source of vertigo.
- The vestibuloocular reflex differentiates between a central and peripheral lesion (abnormal in a peripheral lesion).
- Acute vertigo and deafness may indicate a pontocerebellar lesion.

TABLE 7.1. VERTIGO AND OTOLOGIC EMERGENCIES

Diagnosis	Clues	Therapy
Herpes zoster oticus	Ear lobe vesicles, hearing loss, facial palsy	Acyclovir 10–12 mg/kg IV every 8 hours for 10 days
Bacterial labyrinthitis	Acute deafness, prior cholesteatoma, meningitis	Surgical management or specific antibiotics
Malignant external otitis	Extreme ear pain, facial palsy (*Pseudomonas aeruginosa*)	Ciprofloxacin 750 mg orally twice daily or gentamicin 1.7 mg/kg/dose every 8 hours
Perilymph fistula	Tinnitus, hearing loss, position vertigo, prior strain or valsalva or barotrauma	Conservative first, then surgery
Labyrinth hemorrhage	Nausea, vomiting, hearing loss, trauma	Correct coagulopathy

Data from Cummings CW, Fredrickson JM, Harker LA, et al. *Otolaryngology*, 3rd ed. St. Louis: Mosby, 1998. With permission of the publisher.

TABLE 7.2. NYSTAGMUS IN ACUTE LESIONS OF THE CENTRAL VESTIBULAR SYSTEM

Type	Features	Lesion
Downbeat	Increasing amplitude with downgaze	Cervicomedullary junction
Upbeat	Increasing amplitude with upgaze	Paramedian medulla oblongata or brainstem
Rebound	With continuous lateral position, reversal or disappearance	Cerebellum
Dissociated	Disconjugate	Brainstem
Bobbing	Downward jerk with slow return to midposition	Pons

TABLE 7.3. CLINICAL SIGNS DIFFERENTIATING CENTRAL (BRAINSTEM-CEREBELLUM) FROM PERIPHERAL (VESTIBULAR)

Sign	Peripheral	Central
Spontaneous	Horizontal torsional	Pure horizontal
Nystagmus	Suppressed with visual fixation	Pure vertical
Smooth pursuit	Intact	Broken
Positional nystagmus	Delay, fatigability	No delay or fatigability

Adapted from Seemungal BM, Bronstein AM. A practical approach to acute vertigo. *Pract Neurol* 2008; 8:211–221. With permission of the publisher.

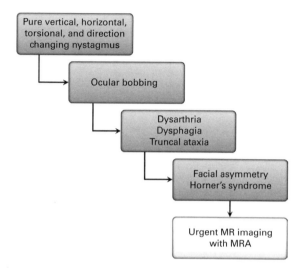

Figure 7.2: Critical steps in vertigo evaluation due to a lesion in the central nervous system.

MR, magnetic resonance; MRA, magnetic resonance angiography.

Chapter 8

Moving, Jerking, and Spasm

PRACTICAL NOTES

- Acute movement disorders may be drug-induced or a result of intoxications.
- Acute catatonia is a life-threatening disorder that requires immediate treatment of its dysautonomic features.
- Chorea can be a first manifestation of a systemic medical illness.
- Acute myoclonus may be the first manifestation of a serotonin syndrome and more common due to increased use in SSRIs

TABLE 8.1. DRUGS CAUSING
MYOCLONUS

Drug Type	Drug
Antidepressants	Monoamine oxidase inhibitors
	Tricyclic antidepressants
	Lithium
	Fluoxetine
Antimicrobials	Penicillin
	Ticarcillin
	Carbenicillin
	Cephalosporins
	Acyclovir
	Isoniazid
Anesthetics	Etomidate
	Enflurane
	Isoflurane
	Fentanyl
	Anticonvulsants
	Valproic acid
	Carbamazepine
	Clozapine
	Vigabatrin
Calcium channel-blocking agents	Verapamil
	Nifedipine
	Diltiazem
	Amlodipine

Opiate derivatives	Meperidine
	Methadone
	Morphine
	Oxycodone
	Other drugs
	Bismuth
	Chlorambucil
Overdoses or poisonings	Antihistamines
	Methyl bromide fumes
	Organic mercury
	Gasoline sniffing
	Dichloromethane
	Strychnine
	Chloralose (rodenticide)

Source: Adapted from reference 23.

TABLE 8.2. DRUG-INDUCED DYSTONIA

Anesthetics
Antiepileptics
Benzodiazepines
Calcium antagonists
Dextromethorphan
Dopamine agonists
Metoclopramide
Monoamine oxidase inhibitors
Ondansetron
Ranitidine
Selective serotonin reuptake inhibitors
Sumatriptan
Amitriptyline

TABLE 8.3. DRUG-INDUCED CHOREA

Amphetamines
Cocaine
Pemoline
Oral contraceptives
Tricyclic antidepressants
Selective serotonin reuptake inhibitors
Theophylline
Lithium
Antiepileptics

TABLE 8.4. DRUG-INDUCED TREMORS

Antiepileptics
Antidepressants
Antihyperglycemics
Calcium channel blockers
Corticosteroids
Dopamine receptor–blocking agents
Lithium
Theophylline
Thyroxine

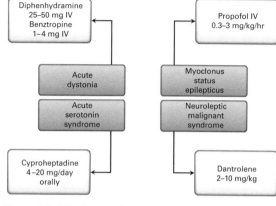

Figure 8.2: The four major acute movement disorders and initial therapy.

IV, intravenous.

Part III Evaluation of Presenting Symptoms Indicating Critical Emergency

Chapter 9

Can't Walk or Stand

PRACTICAL NOTES

- Acute gait disorder may be caused by viral infections or recent vaccination in children and acute cerebellar infarction or medication overdose in the elderly.
- Acute paraplegia may be a consequence of spinal cord compression, and neuroimaging with MRI is urgently needed.
- Acute chest pain and paraplegia requires immediate evaluation for aortic dissection.

TABLE 9.1. ACUTE OR SUBACUTE ATAXIA

Intoxications and poisonings

Acute occlusion of PICA

Acute demyelination or multiple sclerosis

Acute cerebellar ataxia*

(vaccinations, varicella zoster virus)

Normal pressure hydrocephalus

Paraneoplastic disease

---

*Children usually less than 5 years old. PICA, posterior inferior cerebellar artery.

TABLE 9.2. ACUTE PARAPLEGIA

Disorder	History	Suggest
Myelitis	Vaccination	Postvaccination myelopathy
	Febrile illness	Postinfectious transverse myelitis
	Optic neuritis	Multiple sclerosis or Devic disease
	Travel	Schistosomiasis, cysticercosis
	Tick bite	Lyme disease
	Immunosuppression, AIDS	Tuberculosis, aspergillosis, coccidioidomycosis, syphilis
Myelopathy	Cancer	Acute necrotic myelopathy
	Aortic aneurysms or recent catheterization, low back pain	Infarction of the cord (thromboemboli, fibrocartilaginous emboli)
	Connective tissue disease (Sjögren syndrome, SLE)	Vasculitis
	Cancer	Radiation myelopathy
		Paraneoplastic myelopathy
	Anticoagulation	Epidural hematoma
	Progressive symptoms with occasional exacerbation, profound muscle wasting	Intramedullary hemorrhage
		Spinal AVM
		Dural AV fistula

Polyradiculopathy	Diarrhea, URI, CMV, HSV, EBV, diabetes mellitus, leukemia, sarcoidosis	Guillain-Barré syndrome Acute diabetic polyradiculopathy
Neoplastic meningitis	Carcinoma, lymphoma, or other hematologic-oncologic disease	Leptomeningeal spread
Neuromuscular junction disorders	Dysphagia, diplopia, ptosis, fatigability, small cell lung cancer Dry mouth; sixth nerve palsy; fixed, dilated pupils	Myasthenia gravis Lambert-Eaton syndrome Botulism
Myopathy	Autoimmune disorder Malar, perioral skin rash Exercise intolerance and myoglobinuria Periodic attacks (minutes to hours) Thyrotoxicosis	Polymyositis Dermatomyositis Metabolic myopathy Hyperkalemia or hypokalemic paralysis Hypokalemic paralysis

AIDS, acquired immunodeficiency syndrome; AV, arteriovenous; AVM, arteriovenous malformation; CMV, cytomegalovirus; EBV, Epstein-Barr virus; HSV, herpes simplex virus; SLE, systemic lupus erythematosus; URI, upper respiratory infection.

TABLE 9.3. ACUTE SPINAL CORD SYNDROMES

Complete

All sensory modalities and reflexes impaired below
    level of severance: pinprick loss most valuable
Flaccid, paraplegia, or tetraplegia
Fasciculations
Urinary or rectal sphincter dysfunction
Sweating, piloerection diminished below lesions
Genital reflexes lost, priapism

Central

Vest-like loss of pain and temperature
Initial sparing of proprioception
Sacral sensation spared
Paraparesis or tetraparesis

Hemisection

Loss of pain and temperature opposite to the lesion
Sensory loss two segments below lesion
Loss of proprioception on same side as lesion
Light touch may be normal or minimally decreased
Weakness on same side as lesion

Anterior

Pain and temperature loss below lesion
Proprioception spared
Flaccid, areflexia
Paraparesis or tetraparesis
Fasciculations
Urinary or rectal sphincter dysfunction

CAPSULE 9.1   LOCALIZING SPINAL CORD LESIONS

FORAMEN MAGNUM SYNDROME AND LESIONS OF THE UPPER CERVICAL CORD

- Suboccipital pain and neck stiffness, Lhermitte sign, occipital and fingertip paresthesias
- Sensory dissociation may be present.
- Sensory findings of posterior column dysfunction may be present.
- High cervical compressive findings (spastic tetraparesis, long-tract sensory findings, bladder disturbance)
- Lower cranial nerve palsies (CN IX–XII) may occur from regional extension of the pathologic process.
- Lesions affecting the C5 segment may compromise the diaphragm.
- With C5 segment lesions, biceps and brachioradialis reflexes are absent or diminished, whereas the triceps reflex and the finger flexor reflex are exaggerated (because of corticospinal tract compression at C5).
- With C6 segment lesions, biceps, brachioradialis, and triceps reflexes are diminished or absent but the finger flexor reflex (C8–T1) is exaggerated.

(continued)

CAPSULE 9.1 (CONTINUED)

LESIONS OF THE SEVENTH CERVICAL SEGMENT

- Paresis involves flexors and extensors of the wrists and fingers.
- Biceps and brachioradialis reflexes are preserved, and the finger flexor reflex is exaggerated.
- May result in flexion of the forearm following olecranon tap. (Weakness of the triceps prevents its contraction and elbow extension, whereas muscles innervated by normal segments above the lesion are allowed to contract.)
- Sensory loss at and below the third and fourth digits (including medial arm and forearm) is present.

LESIONS OF THE EIGHTH CERVICAL AND FIRST THORACIC SEGMENTS

- Weakness that predominantly involves the small hand muscles with associated spastic paraparesis
- With C8 lesions, the triceps reflex (C6–C8) and finger flexor reflex (C8–T1) are decreased.
- With T1 lesions, the triceps reflex is preserved, but the finger flexor reflex is decreased.
- Unilateral or bilateral Horner syndrome is possible with C8–T1 lesions.
- Sensory loss involves the fifth digit, medial forearm and arm, and the rest of the body below the lesion.

LESIONS OF THE THORACIC SEGMENTS

- Root pain or paresthesias that mimic intercostal neuralgia
- Segmental lower motor neuron involvement is difficult to detect clinically.
- Paraplegia, sensory loss below thoracic level, and bowel and bladder disturbances occur.
- With a lesion above T5, vasomotor control may be impaired.
- With a lesion at the T10 level, upper abdominal musculature is preserved but lower abdominal muscles are weak. For example, when the head is flexed against resistance with the patient supine, the intact upper abdominal muscles pull the umbilicus upward (Beevor sign).
- If the lesion lies above T6, superficial abdominal reflexes are present.
- If the lesion is at or below T10, upper and middle abdominal reflexes are present.
- If the lesion is below T12, all abdominal reflexes are present.

LESIONS OF THE FIRST LUMBAR SEGMENT

- Weakness in all muscles of the lower extremities; lower abdominal muscle paresis
- Sensory loss includes both the lower extremities up to the level of the groin and the back to a level above the buttocks.
- With long-standing lesions, the patellar and ankle jerks are brisk.

(continued)

CAPSULE 9.1 (CONTINUED)

LESIONS OF THE SECOND LUMBAR SEGMENT

- Spastic paraparesis but no weakness of abdominal musculature
- Cremasteric reflex (L2) is not elicitable, and patellar jerk may be depressed.
- Ankle jerks are hyperactive.

LESIONS OF THE THIRD LUMBAR SEGMENT

- Some preservation of hip flexion (iliopsoas and sartorius) and leg adduction (adductor longus, pectineus, and gracilis).
- Patellar jerks are decreased or not elicitable.
- Ankle jerks are hyperactive.

LESIONS OF THE FOURTH LUMBAR SEGMENT

- Better hip flexion and leg adduction than in L1–L3 lesions
- Knee flexion and leg extension are better performed, and the patient is able to stand by stabilizing the knees.
- Patellar jerks are absent, and ankle jerks are hyperactive.

LESIONS OF THE FIFTH LUMBAR SEGMENT

- Normal hip flexion and adduction and leg extension; patient can extend legs against resistance when extremities are flexed at the hip and knee (normal quadriceps).
- Patellar reflexes are present.
- Ankle jerks are hyperactive.

LESIONS OF THE FIRST SACRAL SEGMENT

- Achilles reflexes are absent, but patellar reflexes are preserved.
- Complete sensory loss over the sole, heel, and outer aspect of the foot and ankle.
- Anesthesia over medial calf, posterior thigh

CONUS MEDULLARIS LESIONS

- Paralysis of the pelvic floor muscles and early sphincter dysfunction
- Disruption of the bladder reflex arc results in autonomous neurogenic bladder characterized by loss of voluntary initiation of micturition, increased residual urine, and absent bladder sensation.
- Constipation

(continued)

CAPSULE 9.1 (CONTINUED)

- Impaired erection and ejaculation
- May have symmetric saddle anesthesia
- Pain is uncommon but may involve thighs, buttocks, and perineum.

CAUDA EQUINA LESIONS

- Early radicular pain in the distribution of the lumbosacral roots due to compression below the L3 vertebral level
- Pain may be unilateral or asymmetric and is increased by the Valsalva maneuver.
- With extensive lesions, flaccid, hypotonic, areflexic paralysis develops, affecting the glutei, posterior thigh muscles, and anterolateral muscles of the leg and foot, resulting in a true peripheral type of paraplegia.
- Sensory testing reveals asymmetric sensory loss in saddle region, involving anal, perineal, and genital regions and extending to the dorsal aspect of the thigh, anterolateral aspect of the leg, and outer aspect of the foot.
- Achilles reflexes are absent, and patellar reflexes are variable in response.

- Sphincter changes are similar to those with a conus lesion, but occurrence tends to be late in the clinical course.

- Although it can be concluded that lesions of the conus result in early sphincter compromise, late pain, and symmetric sensory manifestations, whereas cauda lesions have early pain, late sphincter manifestations, and asymmetric sensory findings, this distinction is difficult to establish and is of little practical value.

Source: Data abstracted from The localization of lesions affecting the spinal cord. In Brazis PW, Masdue JC, Biller J, eds. Localization in Clinical Neurology Sixth edition. Philadelphia, Lippincot Williams and Wilkins 2011.

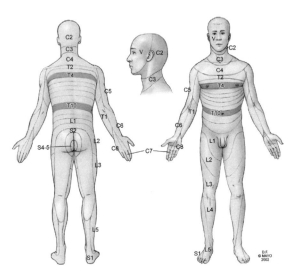

Figure 9.1: Sensory dermatomes.

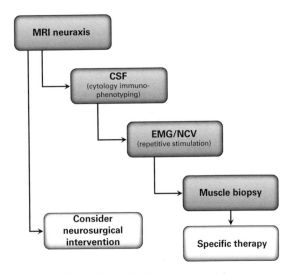

Figure 9.2: Critical steps in the evaluation of gait abnormalities or paraparesis.

CSF, cerebrospinal fluid; EMG/NCV, electromyography/nerve conduction velocity; MRI, magnetic resonance imaging.

Chapter 10

Short of Breath

PRACTICAL NOTES

- Initial appropriate airway management includes mask ventilation with oxygen (10 to 15 L/min flow) after the jaw is lifted upward to open the airway. An oropharyngeal airway may facilitate mask ventilation.
- Intubation is needed in patients with acute brain injury who cannot protect their airway, as shown by frequent hypoxic episodes; in patients with tachycardia and tachypnea associated with neuromuscular failure (GBS, myasthenia gravis); and in patients with primary pulmonary disease (pulmonary edema or progressive aspiration pneumonitis).
- Clinical features of imminent neuromuscular respiratory failure are restlessness, asynchronous breathing, use of sternocleidomastoid muscles, and forehead sweating. Pulmonary function tests are of potential use; the critical values are vital capacity, 20 mL/kg; maximum inspiratory pressure, −30 cm H_2O; and maximum expiratory pressure, 40 cm H_2O.

TABLE 10.1. THREE MAJOR CAUSES OF RESPIRATORY FAILURE IN ACUTE NEUROLOGIC DISEASE

Abnormal respiratory drive

Sedatives (e.g., opioids, barbiturates, benzodiazepines, propofol)

Pontomedullary lesion (e.g., hemorrhage, infarct, trauma)

Hypercapnia

Hypothermia

Hypothyroidism

Abnormal respiratory conduit

Upper airway obstruction

Massive aspiration

Neurogenic pulmonary edema

Pneumothorax (e.g., after subclavian catheterization)

Abnormal respiratory mechanics

Spinal cord lesion (e.g., trauma, demyelination, amyotrophic lateral sclerosis)

Absent or decreased neuromuscular junction traffic (e.g., myasthenia gravis, organophosphates, botulism, tick paralysis)

Diaphragm failure (e.g., myopathies, phrenic nerve lesion trauma)

TABLE 10.2. CLINICAL FEATURES OF NEUROMUSCULAR RESPIRATORY FAILURE

Restlessness, out of breath sensation

Tachycardia (pulse rate > 100/min)

Tachypnea (respiratory rate > 20/min)

Use of sternocleidomastoid or scalene muscles (by palpation alone)

Forehead sweating

Hesitant, constantly interrupting speech

Asynchronous (paradoxical) breathing

TABLE 10.3. PULMONARY FUNCTION TESTS TO MONITOR NEUROMUSCULAR RESPIRATORY FAILURE

Parameter	Normal Value	Critical Value
Vital capacity	40–70 mL/kg	20 mL/kg
Maximum inspiratory pressure	Male ≥ −100 cm H_2O Female ≥ −70 cm H_2O	−30 cm H_2O
Maximum expiratory pressure	Male > 100 cm H_2O Female > 40 cm H_2O	40 cm H_2O

TABLE 10.4. RAPID SEQUENCE INTUBATION

Preinduction agents	Lidocaine 1.5 mg/kg IV Fentanyl 2–3 µg/kg IV push
Induction agents	Etomidate 0.3 mg/kg IV push Ketamine 2 mg/kg IV push
Paralytic agents	Succinylcholine 1.5 mg/kg IV push Rocuronium 1 mg/kg IV push

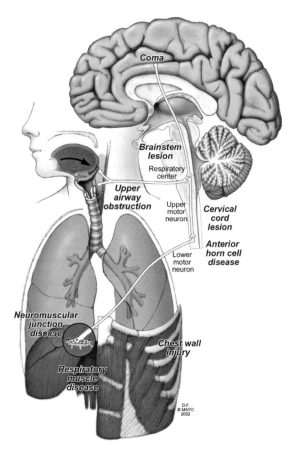

Figure 10.1: Causes of respiratory failure in neurologic disease at different levels of the nervous system.

Seizing

PRACTICAL NOTES

- Different types of status epilepticus require different therapeutic approaches.
- Treatment of tonic-clonic status epilepticus is successful in more than two-thirds of the cases using a combination of adequate doses of IV lorazepam and fosphenytoin.
- Seizure recurrence is substantial in a patient with a new-onset seizure and demonstrable brain lesion and thus requires antiepileptic therapy and often admission.

CHAPTER 11 Seizing

CAPSULE 11.2 ANTIEPILEPTIC DRUGS AND SIDE EFFECTS

PHENYTOIN

Phenytoin is rapidly distributed to body tissue and the brain. Respiratory depression does not occur in loading doses of 10–20 mg/kg. Sinus bradycardia is the most common cardiac arrhythmia. Transient diastolic pauses may occur, and the drug may worsen any heart block. Asystole has been reported. Phenytoin can be mixed only in isotonic saline because it precipitates in glucose. Oral dosage should start 6–12 hours after infusion.

FOSPHENYTOIN

Fosphenytoin sodium (Cerebyx) is a prodrug of phenytoin that is rapidly converted by enzymes to phenytoin.[9] Both intravenous and intramuscular administrations of 15–20 mg PE/kg produced therapeutic total (10–20 mcg/mL) and free (1–2 mcg/mL) plasma levels. Intramuscular loading (9–12 mg/kg phenytoin equivalent) produces therapeutic levels in 1–2 hours and can be considered in status epilepticus but only if intravenous access is not available. Fosphenytoin is completely water soluble. Therefore, phlebitis, hypotension, and cardiac arrhythmias, typically associated with propylene glycol-based intravenous phenytoin, are infrequent. However, cardiac arrhythmias may still occur when fosphenytoin is infused at rates > 150 mg PE/min. There is no pharmacokinetic drug interaction with intravenously administered diazepam or lorazepam. Major side effects are nystagmus, headaches, ataxia, and drowsiness. Previously unrecognized and highly typical side effects (up to 30%) are transient but very annoying paresthesias and itching in the groin, genitalia, and head and neck.

MIDAZOLAM

It is not clear why midazolam works when benzodiazepines fail to control seizures.[5,15,54] The half-life of midazolam (1–12 hours) is less than that of lorazepam (10–12 hours), and midazolam produces sedation of short duration in status epilepticus. Hourly infusion of 0.1–0.6 mg/kg should be continued for at least 12 hours before the dose is tapered. The cost, comparable with that of lorazepam, is high, approaching $800 for 24 hours of continuous infusion. The absence of propylene glycol solution in midazolam reduces the risk of hypotension, bradycardia, and electrocardiographic changes, which are more common with diazepam and lorazepam. High rates of infusion may produce cardiac depression and hypotension.[26] Often, the mean dose to abolish seizure activity is three times the starting dose.

PROPOFOL

Propofol has been considered controversial because of its association with myoclonic jerking and opisthotonos in humans. However, several studies have confirmed that it inhibits seizure activity.

(continued)

CAPSULE 11.2 CONTINUED

Propofol has been used in anesthetic doses to control status epilepticus and has reduced the risk of prolonged seizures in electroconvulsive therapy. A bolus of propofol may cause significant hypotension and is ill-advised. Bradycardia, hypotension, and lactic acidosis are side effects. Propofol infusion syndrome (acute hypotension, sudden cardiac arrest, metabolic acidosis) is rare but more common in patients with acute neurologic disease and prolonged infusions of high doses.

BARBITURATES

Phenobarbital is much more potent than pentobarbital. Its major drawbacks are direct myocardial depression and vascular dilatation, but these are not treatment-limiting. Phenobarbital also has a very long elimination half-life (24–140 hours) but zero-order elimination at high doses (constant amount of drug elimination per unit of time). Intravenous pentobarbital (1–3 mg/kg/hr) virtually always controls status epilepticus, usually preceded by electrographic recurrence of seizure activity. Use of this drug nearly always requires vasopressors to maintain adequate blood pressures.

TABLE 11.1. CAUSES OF CONVULSIVE STATUS EPILEPTICUS

Change in antiepileptic drugs
Bacterial meningitis or intracranial abscess
Encephalitis
Intracranial tumor or metastasis
Stroke
Arteriovenous malformation
Withdrawal of benzodiazepines
Drugs or alcohol withdrawal
Hyperglycemia
Hypoglycemia
Hyponatremia
Preeclampsia

TABLE 11.2. DIAGNOSTIC TESTS IN A PATIENT WITH DE NOVO SEIZURE IN ED

Computed tomographic scan with contrast *
Cervical spine radiograph (if trauma is suspected)
Cerebrospinal fluid (predominantly in
    immunosuppressed patients, human
    immunodeficiency virus)
Toxicologic screen, alcohol level
Sodium, calcium, magnesium, blood urea nitrogen,
    creatinine, complete white blood cell count,
    glucose

* if feasible, MRI

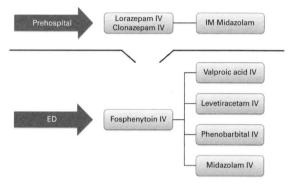

Figure 11.4: Algorithm for initial management of convulsive status epilepticus.

IV, intravenous.

Chapter 12

Comatose

PRACTICAL NOTES

- Neurologic examination followed by categorization in bihemispheric, brainstem displacement or intrinsic brainstem injury may be helpful in the focused assessment and evaluation of coma.
- Early stabilizing of the comatose patient may include intubation for airway protection, correction of hypotension and hypovolemia, and correction of acute metabolic derangements.
- Early recognition of increased ICP from mass effect or acute hydrocephalus is essential, and early medical and surgical intervention may reduce morbidity.
- Intoxications are common causes of coma in the ED, and drug screens are mandatory, followed by specific antidotes if indicated.

TABLE 12.1. CLASSIFICATION AND MAJOR CAUSES OF COMA

Structural Brain Injury	*Cerebellum (with displacement of brainstem)*
Hemisphere	Cerebellar infarct
Unilateral (with displacement)	Cerebellar hematoma
Intraparenchymal hematoma	Cerebellar abscess
Middle cerebral artery occlusion	Cerebellar glioma
Hemorrhagic contusion	
Cerebral abscess	***Acute Metabolic-Endocrine Derangement***
Brain tumor	Hypoglycemia
	Hyperglycemia (nonketotic hyperosmolar)
Bilateral	Hyponatremia
Penetrating traumatic brain injury	Hypernatremia
Multiple traumatic brain contusions	Addison's disease
Anoxic-ischemic encephalopathy	Hypercalcemia
Aneurysmal subarachnoid hemorrhage	Acute hypothyroidism
Multiple cerebral infarcts	Acute panhypopituitarism
Bilateral thalamic infarcts	Acute uremia
Cerebral venous thrombosis	Hyperbilirubinemia
Lymphoma	

Encephalitis
Gliomatosis
Acute disseminated encephalomyelitis
Cerebral edema
Multiple brain metastases
Acute hydrocephalus
Acute leukoencephalopathy

Brainstem

Pontine hemorrhage
Basilar artery occlusion
Central pontine myelinolysis
Brainstem hemorrhagic contusion

Hypercapnia

Diffuse Physiologic Brain Dysfunction

Generalized tonic-clonic seizures
Poisoning, illicit drug use
Hypothermia
Gas inhalation
Acute (lethal) catatonia, malignant neuroleptic syndrome

Psychogenic Unresponsiveness

Hysterical
Malingering

TABLE 12.2. IMPORTANT SKIN ABNORMALITIES THAT MAY HAVE DISCRIMINATORY VALUE IN THE ASSESSMENT OF COMA

Sign or Symptom	Meaning
Acne	Long-term antiepileptic drug use
Bullae	Barbiturates, sedative-hypnotic drugs
Butterfly eruption on face	Systemic lupus erythematosus
Cold, malar flush, yellow tinge, puffy face	Myxedema
Dark pigmentation	Addison's disease
Dryness	Barbiturate poisoning, anticholinergic agents
Edema	Acute renal failure
Purpura	Meningococcal meningitis, thrombotic thrombocytopenic purpura, vasculitis, disseminated intravascular coagulation, aspirin intoxication
Rash	Meningitis or seasonal encephalitis
Sweating	Cholinergic poisoning, hypoglycemia, sympathomimetics, malignant catatonia or acute paroxysmal sympathetic hyperactivity, thyroid storm

TABLE 12.3. COMMON CHANGES IN VITAL SIGNS IN COMA FROM POISONING

Toxin	Blood Pressure	Pulse	Respiration	Temperature	Additional Signs
Amphetamines	↑	↑	↑	↑	Mydriasis
Arsenic	→	↑	?	?	Marked dehydration
Barbiturates	→	?	→	→	Bullae, hypoglycemia
β-adrenergic blockers	→	→	?	?	Seizures
Carbon monoxide	?	?	?	?	Seizures
Cocaine	↑	↑	?	↑	Mydriasis, seizures
Cyclic antidepressants	→	↑	?	↑	Mydriasis
Ethylene glycol	?	↑	↑	?	Anion gap and osmolar gap, metabolic acidosis
Lithium	→	?	?	?	Seizures, myoclonus
Methanol	→	?	→	?	Anion gap and osmolar gap, acidosis

(continued)

TABLE 12.3. (CONTINUED)

Opioids	→	→	→	Miosis
Organophosphates	→	↓/↑	↑/↓	~	Fasciculations, bronchospasm, hypersalivation, sweating, miosis
Phencyclidine	↑	↑	~	↑	Miosis, myoclonus
Phenothiazine	→	↑	~	↓/↑	Dystonia
Salicylates	~	~	↑	↑	Anion gap, metabolic acidosis, respiratory alkalosis
Sedative-hypnotics	→	~	→	→	Bullae

↑ = increase; ↓ = decrease; ~ = no change

TABLE 12.4. GLASGOW COMA SCALE

Eye opening

4 Spontaneous
3 To speech
2 To pain
1 None

Best motor response

6 Obeying
5 Localizing pain
4 Withdrawal
3 Abnormal flexing
2 Extensor response
1 None

Best verbal response

5 Oriented
4 Confused conversation
3 Inappropriate words
2 Incomprehensible sounds
1 None

TABLE 12.6. Laboratory Values Compatible with Coma in Patients with Acute Metabolic and Endocrine Derangements*

Derangement	Serum
Hyponatremia	≤ 110 mmol/L
Hypernatremia	≥ 160 mmol/L
Hypercalcemia	≥ 15 mg/dL
Hypermagnesemia	≥ 5 mg/dL
Hypercapnia	≥ 70 mm Hg
Hypoglycemia	≤ 40 mg/dL
Hyperglycemia	≥ 800 mg/dL

* Sudden decline in value is obligatory.

TABLE 12.7. Frequent Abnormalities on Neuroimaging Studies in Coma

Findings	Suggested Disorders
Computed Tomography	
Mass lesion	Hematoma, hemorrhagic contusion, MCA territory infarct
Hemorrhage in basal cisterns	Aneurysmal SAH
Intraventricular hemorrhage	Arteriovenous malformation
Multiple hemorrhagic infarcts	Cerebral venous thrombosis
Multiple cerebral infarcts	Endocarditis, coagulopathy, CNS vasculitis
Diffuse cerebral edema	Cardiac arrest, fulminant meningitis, acute hepatic necrosis, encephalitis
Acute hydrocephalus	Aqueduct obstruction, colloid cyst, pineal region tumor
Pontine or cerebellum hemorrhage	Hypertension, arteriovenous malformation, cavernous malformation
Shear lesions in the white matter	Traumatic brain injury

Magnetic Resonance Imaging

Bilateral caudate and putaminal lesions	Carbon monoxide poisoning, methanol
Hyperdense signal along sagittal, straight, and transverse sinuses	Cerebral venous thrombosis
Lesions in corpus callosum, white matter	Traumatic head injury
Diffuse confluent hyperintense lesions in white matter	Acute disseminated encephalomyelitis, immunosuppressive agent or chemotherapeutic agent toxicity, metabolic leukodystrophies
Pontine trident-shaped lesion	Central pontine myelinolysis
Thalamus, occipital, pontine lesions	Acute basilar artery occlusion
Temporal, frontal lobe hyperintensities	Herpes simplex encephalitis

CNS, central nervous system; MCA, middle cerebral artery; SAH, subarachnoid hemorrhage.

TABLE 12.8. BLOOD GAS ABNORMALITIES DUE TO TOXINS

Metabolic Acidosis (Anion Gap)	*Respiratory Acidosis*
Methanol	Barbiturates
Ethanol	Benzodiazepines
Paraldehyde	Botulism toxin
Isoniazid	Opioids
Salicylates	Strychnine
Metabolic Alkalosis	Tetrodotoxin
Diuretics	*Respiratory Alkalosis*
Nonketotic hyperglycemia	Salicylates
Lithium	Amphetamines
	Anticholinergics
	Cocaine
	Cyanide
	Paraldehyde
	Theophylline
	Carbon monoxide

TABLE 12.9. LABORATORY TESTS IN THE EVALUATION OF COMA

Hematocrit, white blood cell count

Glucose

Electrolytes

Urea, creatinine

Aspartate transaminase (AST) and
γ-glutamyltransferase (GGT)

Ammonia

Osmolality

Arterial blood gases (optional)

Platelets, smear, fibrinogen degradation products,
international normalized ratio (optional)

Plasma thyrotropin (optional)

Blood and cerebrospinal fluid cultures (optional)

Toxic screen in blood and urine (optional)

Cerebrospinal fluid (protein, cells, glucose, India
ink stain, and cryptococcal antigen, viral titers)
(optional)

90

TABLE 12.10. MANAGEMENT
OF ACUTE SUPRATENTORIAL MASS
WITH BRAIN SHIFT

Stabilizing Measures
Intubation and mechanical ventilation
Correct hypoxemia with O_2 nasal catheter, 3–4 L/
    min, or face mask
Elevate head to 30 degrees
Treat extreme agitation with lorazepam, 2 mg IV, or
    propofol, 0.3 mg/kg/hr IV
Correct coagulopathy with fresh-frozen plasma,
    vitamin K (if applicable), PCC or factor VIIa

Specific Medical Measures
Hyperventilation: increase respiratory rate to 20
    breaths/minute, aim at $PaCO_2$ of 25–30 mm Hg
Mannitol 20%, 1 g/kg; if no effect, 2 g/kg; aim at
    plasma osmolality of 310 mOsm/L
Dexamethasone, 100 mg intravenously (in tumors
    only)

Specific Surgical Measures
Evacuation of hematoma
Placement of drain in abscess
Decompressive craniectomy with brain swelling

$PaCO_2$, partial arterial pressure of CO_2; IV, intravenously; PCC,
    prothrombin complex concentrate.

TABLE 12.11. MANAGEMENT OF ACUTE SUBTENTORIAL MASS OR BRAINSTEM LESION

Stabilizing Measures
Intubation and mechanical ventilation
Correct hypoxemia with 3 L of O_2/min
Flat body position (in acute basilar artery occlusion)
Specific Medical Measures
Intra-arterial tPA (in basilar artery occlusion)
Mannitol 20%, 1 g/kg (in acute cerebellar mass)
Hyperventilation to $PaCO_2$ of 25–50 mm Hg (in acute cerebellar mass)
Specific Surgical Measures
Ventriculostomy
Suboccipital craniectomy

$PaCO_2$, partial arterial pressure of CO_2.

TABLE 12.12. EMPIRICAL ANTIBIOTIC AND ANTIVIRAL THERAPY IN PATIENTS IN COMA ASSOCIATED WITH INFLAMMATORY CONDITIONS

Antibacterial	Cefotaxime 2 g every 6 hours; Vancomycin 20 mg/kg IV every 12 hours for target trough level at 15–20 mcg/mL
Antiviral	Acyclovir 10 mg/kg every 8 hours
Antiparasitic	Pyrimethamine 50–75 mg per day orally
	Sulfadiazine 2–8 g orally divided every 6 hours
	Praziquantel 75 mg/kg/day orally in 3 divided doses

TABLE 12.13. DIFFERENTIAL DIAGNOSIS
IN FAILURE TO REVERSE COMA
FROM ALLEGED OPIATE OVERDOSE

Traumatic brain injury

Hypoglycemia

Anoxic–ischemic encephalopathy

Mixed overdose with drug in another category
(e.g., cocaine, ethanol)

Central nervous system infection, systemic
infection, sepsis

Seizures, nonconvulsive status epilepticus (rare)

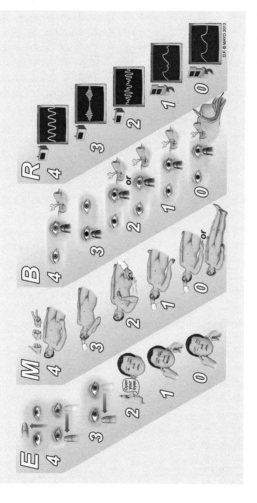

(continued)

Figure 12.3: The FOUR Score.

Eye response

4 = eyelids open or opened, tracking, or blinking to command

3 = eyelids open but not tracking

2 = eyelids closed but open to loud voice

1 = eyelids closed but open to pain

0 = eyelids remain closed with pain

Motor response

4 = thumbs-up, fist, or peace sign

3 = localizing to pain

2 = flexion response to pain

1 = extension response to pain

0 = no response to pain or generalized myoclonus status

Brainstem reflexes

4 = pupil and corneal reflexes present

3 = one pupil wide and fixed

2 = pupil or corneal reflexes absent

1 = pupil and corneal reflexes absent

0 = pupil, corneal, and cough reflexes absent

Respiration

4 = not intubated, regular breathing

3 = not intubated, Cheyne-Stokes breathing

2 = not intubated, irregular breathing

1 = breathes above ventilatory rate

0 = breathes at ventilator rate or apnea

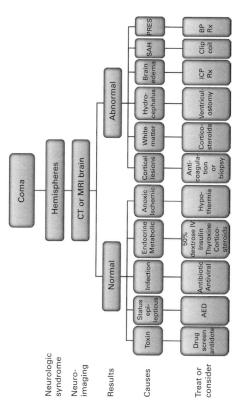

Figure 12.9: Algorithm to elucidate cause of coma based on bihemispheric signs.

AED, antiepileptic drugs; BP, blood pressure; CT, computed tomography; HEP, heparin; ICP, intracranial pressure; IV, intravenous; MRI, magnetic resonance imaging; PRES, posterior reversible encephalopathy syndrome; RX, treatment; SAH, subarachnoid hemorrhage; TBI, traumatic brain injury.

From Wijdicks EFM. *The Comatose Patient*. 2nd edition. New York: Oxford University Press, 2014.

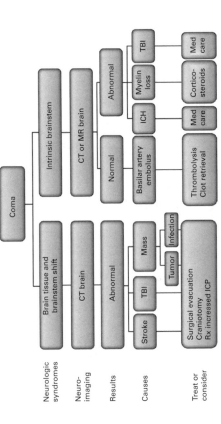

Figure 12.10: Algorithm to elucidate cause of coma based on brainstem displacement and intrinsic brainstem signs.

CT, computed tomography; ICH, intracranial hemorrhage; ICP, intracranial pressure; MR, magnetic resonance; TBI, traumatic brain injury.

From Wijdicks EFM. *The Comatose Patient*. 2nd edition. New York: Oxford University Press, 2014.

Chapter 15

General Perspectives of Care

PRACTICAL NOTES

- Alignment of the body is monitored daily: arms flexed, hands on pillows, and trochanter rolls in place. Compression points are monitored for development of erythema or early decubital ulcers.
- Incentive spirometry (every 2 hours; 6 trials during the day) is begun in patients with neuromuscular respiratory failure and after craniotomy.
- The number of passages during bronchial suctioning must be limited. Evidence of further increase in intracranial pressure should be followed by muting of the response with lidocaine spayed endotracheally
- Requirements for intrahospital transport are stable vital signs for 1 hour, adequate oxygen saturation, and absence of recent seizures. For patients at risk, albumin 5%, mannitol infusion, and anticonvulsants are prepared for possible use during transport.
- Categories of isolation (Centers for Disease Control and Prevention) are strict control, contact isolation, respiratory isolation, tuberculosis isolation, and specific disease isolation precautions (hepatitis, acquired immunodeficiency syndrome).
- Time is taken for detailed communication with the family. Outcome expectations should be explained early, and the purpose of level of care should be clear stated.

TABLE 15.1. ESSENTIALS OF CHEST PHYSIOTHERAPY

Percussion and vibration

Coughing exercises (huffing techniques, oropharyngeal stimulation)

Suctioning (preceded by hyperoxygenation, FiO2 1.0, for 15 seconds)

Mucolytic agents, bronchodilators, and nebulizers for humidification

TABLE 15.2. RECOMMENDATIONS FOR DEEP VEIN THROMBOSIS PROPHYLAXIS

Procedure or Diagnosis	Acute Prophylaxis
Polytrauma	Retrievable filter
Craniotomy (general)	Intermittent pneumatic compression device + graduated compression stockings
Craniotomy (malignancy)	Low-dose unfractionated heparin or low-molecular-weight heparin
Acute spinal cord injury	Low-molecular-weight heparin or low-dose unfractionated heparin

Source: Data from Geerts WH, Bergqvist D, Pineo GF, et al. Prevention of venous thromboembolism: American College of Chest Physicians Evidence based Clinical Practice Guidelines. *Chest* 2008;133:381S–453S.

TABLE 15.3. SUBCUTANEOUS HEPARIN OR LOW-MOLECULAR-WEIGHT HEPARIN

Low risk 48 hours after cerebral hemorrhage
Low risk 24 hours after ischemic stroke
Low risk 12 hours after brain tumor surgery
High risk in unsecured aneurysm
High risk in early traumatic brain injury
Low risk in ventriculostomy (once placed)

TABLE 15.4. PRECAUTIONS BEFORE IN-HOSPITAL TRANSPORT

Minimum of two persons including neurosciences nurse
Stable vital signs for 1 hour
Tracheal suctioning before transport
Patency of intravenous sites checked
Stable vital signs after manual bagging of the patient for several minutes
$SaO_2 > 90\%$
No recent seizures
Mannitol infusion prepared if needed
When indicated, supplies such as antiepileptic drugs (lorazepam 4 mg)
Sufficient supply of administered fluids and drips
Monitor connected for arterial blood pressure tracings and electrocardiography
Defibrillator

TABLE 15.5. ISOLATION CATEGORIES AND EXAMPLES OF INFECTIOUS DISEASES IN EACH CATEGORY

Category	Requirements
Strict isolation	Private room
Rabies	Negative-pressure ventilation
Varicella	Masks, gowns, and gloves at all times
Hemorrhagic fever	Handwashing after glove removal
Contact isolation	Private room
Adenovirus	Mask when close to patient
Herpes simplex (disseminated)	Gowns if soiling likely
Major staphylococcal infections	Gloves for touching infectious material
	Handwashing after glove removal
Respiratory isolation	Private room
Infectious mononucleosis	Mask when close to patient
	Handwashing
Enteric precautions	Gowns if soiling likely
Enterovirus	Gloves for touching infectious material

Hepatitis A, E
Salmonella
Shigella
Campylobacter
Giardia
Rotavirus

Handwashing after glove removal

Drainage and secretion precautions
Herpes simplex (local)
Localized herpes zoster

Gowns if soiling likely
Gloves for touching infectious material
Handwashing after glove removal

Blood and body fluid precautions
Arbovirus
Cytomegalovirus
Hepatitis B, C, D

Human immunodeficiency virus

Fluid-resistant gowns
Gloves for touching infectious material
Mask and glasses with side shields, goggles, or face shield

Care with needles and sharp instruments

TABLE 15.6. CONVERSATIONS WITH FAMILY

Gather all close members including the person with power of attorney

Spend at least 30 minutes

Have nursing staff, clergy, social work, and other consultants present

Discuss "the big picture"

Discuss what the patient is noticing

Discuss what the patient would want under these circumstances

Discuss current plan

Discuss medical and neurosurgical options

Discuss best estimate of outcome

Discuss timeline of improvement, if any

Discuss code status

Set up follow-up meeting

From Wijdicks EFM, *Communicating Prognosis* (New York: Oxford University Press, 2014) .

Chapter 16

Agitation and Pain

PRACTICAL NOTES

- Agitation in a patient with an acute neurologic disorder may be from drug or alcohol withdrawal delirium.
- Alcohol-related delirium is best initially treated with repeated doses of intravenous lorazepam 2 mg.
- Extremely agitated patients are best treated with intravenous lorazepam 1–2 mg, given slowly; haloperidol 5 mg intramuscularly; midazolam 0.02–0.1 mg/kg/hr; or propofol 0.1–0.6 mg/kg/hr. Dexmedetomidine may become a useful alternative to control agitation.
- Propofol is a useful sedative but there is a growing concern with a so-called propofol infusion syndrome, particularly in patients with acute neurologic disease.
- Pain relief has a high priority in neurologic intensive care, and opiates are invariably effective. The preferred agent in acute CNS disorders is codeine.
- Pain relief in GBS is crucial to its management. The preferred agents are oxycodone or morphine.

TABLE 16.1. CAUSES OF DELIRIUM IN THE NEUROSCIENCES INTENSIVE CARE UNIT

Withdrawal syndromes

Alcohol
Benzodiazepines
Barbiturates
Opioids
Central nervous system stimulants

Drug-induced

Antibiotics
Antiarrhythmic agents
Anticholinergic agents
Antihistamines
ß-blockers
Opioids

Metabolic derangements

Hyponatremia
Hyperosmolar hyperglycemia
Endocrine crises

TABLE 16.2. RIKER SEDATION-AGITATION SCALE (SAS)

7	Dangerous agitation	Pulling at endotracheal tube (ETT), trying to remove catheters, climbing over bedrail, striking at staff, thrashing side-to-side
6	Very agitated	Does not calm despite frequent verbal reminding of limits, requires physical restraints, biting ETT
5	Agitated	Anxious or mildly agitated, attempting to sit up, calms down to verbal instructions
4	Calm and cooperative	Calm, awakens easily, follows commands
3	Sedated	Difficult to arouse, awakens to verbal stimuli or gentle shaking, but drifts off again, follows simple commands
2	Very sedated	Arouses to physical stimuli, but does not communicate or follow commands, may move spontaneously
1	Unarousable	Minimal or no response to noxious stimuli, does not communicate or follow commands

TABLE 16.3. THE RICHMOND AGITATION SEDATION SCALE (RASS)

Scale	Definitions	Description
+4	Combative	Combative, violent, immediate danger to staff
+3	Very agitated	Pulls or removes tubes or catheters; aggressive
+2	Agitated	Frequent purposeful movement, fights ventilator
+1	Restless	Anxious and apprehensive, but movements not aggressive or vigorous
0	Alert and calm	
−1	Drowsy	Not fully alert but has eye opening and eye contact (< 10 s)
−2	Light sedation	Briefly awakens to voice with eye opening and eye contact (< 10 s)
−3	Moderate sedation	Movement or eye opening to voice (but no eye contact)
−4	Deep sedation	No response to voice but movement or eye opening to physical stimulation
−5	Not arousable	No response to voice or physical stimulation

From Ely EW, Truman B, Shintani A, et al. Monitoring sedation status over time in ICU patients: reliability and validity of the Richmond Agitation-Sedation Scale (RASS). *JAMA* 2003;289:2983–2991.

TABLE 16.4. TREATMENT OF THE
EXTREMELY AGITATED PATIENT

Not intubated
Lorazepam, 1–2 mg slowly IV every 4 hours
Haloperidol, 5 mg IM q2–4h
Quetiapine, 25 mg t.i.d
Chlordiazepoxide, 50–100 mg IV or IM b.i.d.

Intubated
Midazolam, IV infusion of 0.02–0.08 mg/kg/hr
Fentanyl, IV infusion 1.5 mcg/kg/hr
Propofol, IV infusion of 0.1–0.6 mg/kg/hr

TABLE 16.5. CRITICAL-CARE PAIN OBSERVATION TOOL (CPOT)

Indicator	Description	Score	
Facial expression	No muscular tension observed	Relaxed, neutral	0
	Presence of frowning, brow lowering, orbit tightening, and levator contraction	Tense	1
	All of the above facial movements plus eyelid tightly closed	Grimacing	2
Body movements	Does not move at all (does not necessarily mean absence of pain)	Absence of movements	0
	Slow, cautious movements, touching or rubbing the pain site, seeking attention through movements	Protection	1
	Pulling tube, attempting to sit up, moving limbs/thrashing, not following commands, striking at staff, trying to climb out of bed	Restlessness	2

Muscle tension		Relaxed	0
Evaluation by passive flexion and extension of upper extremities	No resistance to passive movements	Tense, rigid	1
	Resistance to passive movements	Very tense or rigid	2
	Strong resistance to passive movements, inability to complete them		
Compliance with the ventilator (intubated patients)	Alarms not activated, easy ventilation	Tolerating ventilator	0
	Alarms stop spontaneously	Coughing but tolerating	1
	Asynchrony: blocking ventilation, alarms frequently activated	Fighting ventilator	2
OR	Talking in normal tone or no sound	Talking in normal tone or no sound	0
Vocalization (extubated patients)	Sighing, moaning, crying out, sobbing	Sighing, moaning,	1
		crying out, sobbing	2
Total, range			**0–8**

TABLE 16.6. OPIATES FOR PAIN
MANAGEMENT IN THE
NEUROSCIENCE INTENSIVE
CARE UNIT

Agent	Route	Starting Dose (mg)	Peak Effect (hour)	Duration (hour)
Codeine	IM	30	0.5–1	4–6
	PO	30–60	1.5–2	3–4
Morphine	IM	5	0.5–1	3–5
	PO	15	1.5–2	4

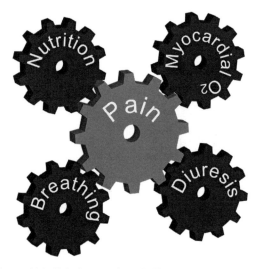

Figure 16.1: Pain has profound effects on physiologic
well-being. Increasing pain causes low tidal volumes,
decreased ventilation, gastric stasis, nausea and
vomiting, poor nutritional intake, hypertension, and
tachycardia and thus increased myocardial oxygen
requirements, and less measurable water and sodium
retention due to an increase in antidiuretic hormone.

Chapter 17

Mechanical Ventilation

PRACTICAL NOTES

- Intubation is needed in patients with acute brain injury who cannot protect their airway, as shown by frequent hypoxic episodes; in patients with tachycardia and tachypnea associated with neuromuscular failure (GBS, myasthenia gravis); and in patients with primary pulmonary disease (pulmonary edema or progressive aspiration pneumonitis).
- A typical order for mechanical ventilation in a stable neurologic patient is IMV, 8–12; FIO_2, 0.4–0.9; tidal volume, 5–10 mL/kg; PEEP, 2–5 cm H_2O; and inspiration-to-expiration ratio, 1:2.
- Noninvasive ventilation (BiPAP) is an option in some patients with neuromuscular respiratory weakness (myasthenia gravis; ALS). It may also function as a possible alternative for intubation in patients with less severe pulmonary disease.
- Tracheostomy may provide better comfort to the patient and facilitates bronchial hygiene. The procedure may reduce length of stay in the NICU. It should be postponed until 2 weeks in patients who can potentially be liberated from the ventilator due to early signs of neurologic improvement.

TABLE 17.1. INDICATION
FOR NONINVASIVE MECHANICAL
VENTILATION (BIPAP) IN NICU

Acute (MG) and chronic neuromuscular disease (ALS)

Coma from intoxications

Weaning mode in extubated patients

Supportive mode following craniotomy

Mild (rapid reversible) exacerbation of COPD and
cardiogenic pulmonary edema

ALS, amyotrophic lateral sclerosis; BiPAP, bilevel positive airway
pressure; COPD, chronic obstructive pulmonary disease. MG,
myasthenia gravis

TABLE 17.2. STARTING NONINVASIVE MECHANICAL VENTILATION (BIPAP)

Set pressures starting with low levels (i.e., pressure support 10 cm H_2O and external PEEP 5 cm H_2O).

When patient is tolerant, tighten straps just enough to avoid major leaks, but not too tight.

Set FIO_2 on ventilator or add low-flow oxygen into the circuit, aiming for $SO_2 > 90\%$.

Set alarms; low pressure alarm should be above PEEP level.

Reset pressures (pressure support increased to get expired tidal volume 6 mL/kg or higher; raise PEEP external to get oxygen saturation 90% or higher).

Consider mild sedation if patient is agitated (e.g., dexmedetomidine 0.15 microgram/kg).

Monitor comfort, respiratory rate, oxygen saturation, and dyspnea every 30 minutes for several hours.

Measure arterial blood gases at baseline and within 2 hours from start.

BiPAP, bilevel positive airway pressure; FIO_2, fraction of inspired oxygen; NIV, noninvasive ventilation; PEEP, positive end-expiratory pressure; SO_2, oxygen saturation.
Adapted from Nava S, Hill N. Noninvasive ventilation in acute respiratory failure. *Lancet* 2000;374:250–259. With permission.

TABLE 17.3. LABORATORY WEANING
CRITERIA IN THE ICU

Measurement	Requirement
PaO_2	> 60 mm Hg
Tidal volume	> 5 mL/kg
Vital capacity	> 15 mL/kg
Minute ventilation	< 10 L/kg
Negative inspiratory pressure	≥ -30 mm Hg

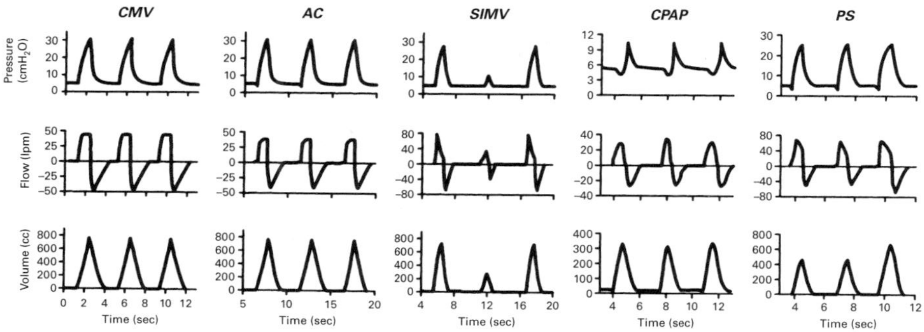

Figure 17.2: Modes of mechanical ventilation. Three breaths with pressure curves and accompanying flow and volume waveforms illustrate the most commonly used selections. CMV (continuous mechanical ventilation): All breaths are machine-generated, and a positive end-expiratory pressure of 5 cm H_2O is evident. AC (assist-control): The first two breaths are patient-triggered, as evidenced by a brief negative deflection in airway pressure followed by a machine-triggered breath. SIMV (synchronized intermittent-mandatory ventilation): Two machine-triggered breaths have a spontaneous breath in between. CPAP (continuous positive airway pressure): All breaths are patient-initiated. PS (pressure support): All breaths are patient-initiated. The waveforms of the volume and flow may vary with each breath but have a common rectangular shape.

Chapter 18

Nutrition

PRACTICAL NOTES

- Energy requirement in the NICU is calculated by the Harris-Benedict formula, and is based on weight, height, and age. Energy expenditure for men = $66.5 + 13.8W + 5H - 6.8A$ and for women = $655 + 9.6W + 1.8H - 4.7A$. Increased caloric needs in critically ill patients may justify a stress factor of 20%.
- Abnormal swallowing during evaluation is characterized by abnormal laryngeal rise, abnormal throat clearing, inefficient coughing, weak tongue protrusion, and abnormal vocal clarity.
- Enteral nutrition with nasogastric or duodenal placement is recommended. Continuous infusion is started at the rate of 25 mL/hr, the rate is gradually increased, and commercially available enteral formulas providing 1 kcal/mL are used.
- PEG is indicated in patients with persistent dysphagia for 2–3 weeks. The procedure can be considered for patients with repeated nasogastric tube extubations, patients with persistent coma from any cause, and patients with a severe brainstem stroke.
- Parenteral nutrition should be initiated in patients who do not tolerate enteral nutrition.

TABLE 18.1. PHYSICAL SIGNS
OF MALNUTRITION

Disorder	Deficiency
Generalized muscle wasting	Any
Easily plucked, thin, dyspigmented hair	Zinc
Nasolabial seborrhea	Any
Fissuring of eyelid corners	Vitamin B$_2$
Angular stomatitis, cheilosis	Vitamin B$_{12}$
Periodontal disease, mottled enamel, and caries	Any
Raw and swollen tongue	Niacin and folate
Spoon-shaped nails	Iron
Hyperkeratosis and petechial hemorrhages of the skin	Vitamin C or K

TABLE 18.2. FEATURES SUGGESTING
ABNORMAL SWALLOWING MECHANISM

Abnormal laryngeal rise
Abnormal throat clearing
Abnormal volitional and reflexive cough
Abnormal gag reflex
Abnormal pharyngeal sensation
Abnormal oral motor rapid movement and strength
Abnormal vocal clarity
Abnormal sipping of water and eating of crackers

TABLE 18.3. FACTORS ALTERING
GASTRIC EMPTYING IN THE
NEUROSCIENCES INTENSIVE CARE UNIT

Diabetes mellitus
Prior vagotomy
Electrolyte abnormalities (e.g., hyperglycemia,
    hypokalemia)
Drugs (opiates, atropine, cephalosporins)
Sepsis or other major systemic infection

TABLE 18.4. COMPLICATIONS
OF ENTERAL FEEDING

Cause	Events
Mechanical	Misplacement
	Tube clogging
	Nasal mucosal ulceration
	Otitis media
	Pharyngitis
	Pneumothorax
	Reflux esophagitis
Gut	Aspiration of stomach contents
	Bloating, constipation
	Diarrhea, vomiting
Metabolic	Liver function abnormalities
	Dehydration
	Hyperglycemia
	Micronutrient deficiency

TABLE 18.5. COMPLICATIONS
OF PERCUTANEOUS ENDOSCOPIC
GASTROSTOMY AND JEJUNOSTOMY
PLACEMENT*

Colocutaneous fistula

Gastric outlet obstruction

Bleeding from submucosal lesions

Ileus

Necrotizing fasciitis

Stoma leakage

Wound and skin infection

Volvulus

*Most complications are minor and occur within the first 3 months
of placement.

Chapter 19

Volume Status and Blood Pressure

PRACTICAL NOTES

- Minimal initial fluid intake in patients with acute brain injury is 200 mL/hr. The goal is a positive fluid balance of approximately 500–750 mL to correct for insensible loss.
- Water deficit in hypovolemic patients can be calculated as follows: 0.6 × body weight × (serum sodium/140)—1 in liters.
- Hypertonic saline 3% has some advantages over albumin and is less costly. Adequate fluid replacement is achieved with sodium chloride 3% at a rate of 4 mL/kg over 3 minutes, or with an immediate bolus of 500 mL of albumin 5%.
- Treatment of hypertension after acute CNS injury is debatable. Treatment is indicated in patients with persistent extreme surges in blood pressure, or impending congestive heart failure.
- Preferred agents for the treatment of hypertension in patients with acute neurologic illness are intravenous labetalol, intravenous nicardipine, or hydralazine.

TABLE 19.1. CLINICAL INDICATORS
OF VOLUME STATUS IN PATIENTS
WITH ACUTE NEUROLOGIC ILLNESS

Urinary output of 1 mL/kg/hr
Fluid intake of 30 mL/kg/day
Fluid balance of 500 to 750 mL/day
Maintenance of body weight
Serum hematocrit
Serum sodium
Creatinine, blood urea nitrogen
Serum glucose
Serum osmolality
Urine osmolality
Urine specific gravity

TABLE 19.2. VOLUME-EXPANDING AGENTS

Agent	Sodium (mEq/L)	Cost*	T½	Side Effects
Isotonic saline	154	D	Minutes	None
Albumin 5%	130–160	20D	5–6 hours	Anaphylaxis, pulmonary edema
Albumin 25%	130–160	20D	5–6 hours	Anaphylaxis, pulmonary edema
Lactated Ringer's solution	130	2D	Minutes	Hypo-osmolar state
Hypertonic saline	513	D	Minutes	Hypernatremia, hyperchloremia, hypokalemia, pulmonary edema
Fresh frozen plasma	170	30D	5–6 hours	Hepatitis, human immunodeficiency virus, anaphylaxis
Dextran 70	154	10D	6 hours	Renal failure, anaphylaxis, pseudohyperglycemia, coagulopathy
Hetastarch	130	10D	12 hours	Coagulopathy, congestive heart failure, vomiting, mild hepatotoxicity

*D is the hospital base price in dollars per purchasing contract. The remaining indicators are compared with this price (e.g., 20D = 20 times more expensive).

TABLE 19.3. BLOOD PRESSURE MANAGEMENT IN ACUTE BRAIN INJURY

Drug	Dose[+]	Action		Adverse Effects	Not Recommended
		Onset	Duration		
Esmolol	500 µg/kg bolus, then infusion of 50–300 mg/kg per min IV	1–2 min	10–30 min	Hypotension, nausea, bronchospasm	Asthma, COPD
Labetalol	20 mg IV bolus, slow 2 min, then every 10 min 40–80 mg injections	5–10 min	3–6 hours	Vomiting, scalp tingling, burning in throat, dizziness, nausea, heart block, liver damage, bronchospasm	Asthma, COPD, ventricular failure
Enalaprilat	0.625 mg IV Slow 5 min, then 1.25 mg q6h	15–30 min	6 hours	Response variable	

(continued)

TABLE 19.3. (CONTINUED)

Drug	Dose†	Action Onset	Duration	Adverse Effects	Not Recommended
Nitroprusside	0.3–10 µg/kg per min as IV infusion	Immediate	3–4 min	Nausea, vomiting, muscle twitching, sweating, thiocyanate intoxication with prolonged use	Coronary artery disease
Diazoxide	1–3 mg/kg (150 mg max dose), repeat 5–15 min	2–4 min	6–12 hours	Nausea, flushing, tachycardia, chest pain	Coronary artery disease
Nicardipine	5 mg/hr infusion IV, to maximum 15 mg/hour	5–10 min	1–4 hours	Tachycardia, headache, flushing	Ventricular failure

| Hydralazine | 10–20 mg IV every 10 min until effect | 10–20 min | 1–4 hours | Tachycardia, flushing, headache | |
| Fenoldopam | 0.1 µg/kg per minute; increase 0.05 µg/kg per min every 15 min until effect | 5–15 min | 1–4 hours | Electrocardiographic changes, reflex tachycardia, hypokalemia, headache | Hepatic cirrhosis |

COPD, chronic obstructive pulmonary disease; min, minutes.

†Ranges given are lowest preferred dose until desired pressure is achieved.

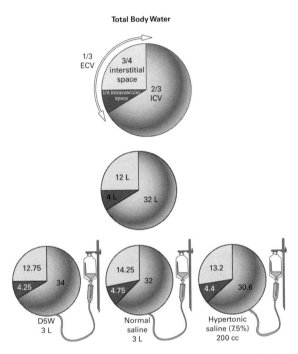

FIGURE 19.1: Body water distribution. Distribution of body water (top) and effect of infusion of different solutions on intravascular volume (bottom).

D5W, 5% dextrose in water; ECV, extracellular volume; ICV, intracellular volume. Note only 200 mL in hypertonic saline and 3 L in other infusions to result in same effect.

Modified from Rainey TG, Read CA. Pharmacology of colloids and crystalloids. In Chernow B, ed., *The Pharmacologic Approach to the Critically Ill Patient*, 3rd ed. Baltimore: Williams & Wilkins, 1994:272–290. With permission of the publisher.

Chapter 20

Anticoagulation and Thrombolysis

PRACTICAL NOTES

- Indications for intravenous heparin in acute ischemic stroke are cardiogenic ischemic stroke –assuming a small territorial stroke, acute carotid or basilar artery occlusion or high-grade critical stenosis, crescendo transient ischemic attacks, and cerebral venous thrombosis.
- Heparin therapy is begun with 80 units/kg intravenously and is continued with 18 units/kg/hr. Activated partial thromboplastin time is determined 6 hours after an initial bolus, and the dose is adjusted.
- When indicated, administration of warfarin (10 mg) can be started on the second day of heparin therapy, and the dose is usually adjusted to an INR of 2.0–3.0. An INR of 3.0–4.5 is recommended in ischemic stroke associated with mechanical prosthetic valves. An INR of 3.0–3.5 is recommended in patients with antiphospholipid antibody syndrome associated with ischemic stroke.
- IV thrombolysis can be considered in patients seen with ischemic stroke with 3 hours of onset. Expansion of the 3-hour time window to 4.5-hour can be considered for most patients.

TABLE 20.1. INDICATIONS FOR INTRAVENOUS HEPARIN IN PATIENTS WITH ACUTE STROKE ADMITTED TO THE NEUROSCIENCE INTENSIVE CARE UNIT

Cardiogenic ischemic stroke

Acute carotid artery occlusion (or high-grade critical stenosis)

Acute basilar artery occlusion (or high-grade critical stenosis)

Crescendo transient ischemic attacks

Cerebral venous thrombosis

TABLE 20.2. WEIGHT-BASED HEPARIN NOMOGRAM*

Start:	Bolus of heparin, 80 units/kg IV		
	Heparin infusion, 18 units/kg/hr (20,000 units in 500 mL of D5W = 40 units/mL)		
Measure:	APTT 6 hours after bolus		
Adjust:	APTT, second	Bolus, U/kg	New infusion rate, U/kg/hr
	< 35	80	22
	35–45	40	20
	46–70	No	18
	71–90	No	16
	> 90	No	15 (stop for 1 hour)

* Some institutions have adopted a low-intensity nomogram (e.g., in ischemic stroke) This includes no loading dose and starts at 12 units/kg/hr.

Administration of warfarin, 10 mg, can be started on the second day of heparin therapy if long-term anticoagulation is warranted. Complete blood cell count with platelet count is done every 3 days. APTT, activated partial thromboplastin time; D5W, 5% dextrose in water.

Modified from Raschke RA, Reilly BM, Guidry JR, et al. The weight-based heparin dosing nomogram compared with a "standard care" nomogram. *Ann Intern Med* 1993;119:874–881. With permission of the American College of Physicians.

TABLE 20.3. INTERNATIONAL NORMALIZED RATIO RECOMMENDATIONS FOR VARIOUS INDICATIONS

Indication	International Normalized Ratio
Prophylaxis of deep vein thrombosis	2.0–3.0
Treatment of venous thrombosis	2.0–3.0
Treatment of pulmonary embolism	2.0–3.0
Atrial fibrillation	2.0–3.0
Tissue heart valve	2.0–3.0
Acute ischemic stroke or transient ischemic attacks	2.0–3.0
Antiphospholipid antibody syndrome	3.0–3.5
Mechanical prosthetic valve	2.5–3.5

Antithrombotic Therapy and Prevention of Thrombosis, 9th ed: American College of Chest Physicians Evidence-Based Clinical Practice Guidelines.
Guyatt GH, Akl EA, Crowther M, Gutterman DD, Schuünemann HJ; American College of Chest Physicians Antithrombotic Therapy and Prevention of Thrombosis Panel. *Chest.* 2012;141(2 Suppl):7S-47S.

TABLE 20.4. COMMONLY USED DRUGS
THAT POTENTIATE OR INTERFERE
WITH THE ACTION OF WARFARIN

Potentiator	Inhibitor
Acetaminophen	Barbiturates
Amiodarone	Carbamazepine
Anesthetics	Chlordiazepoxide
Chloramphenicol	Cholestyramine
Cimetidine	Corticosteroids
Diazoxide	Griseofulvin
Erythromycin	Haloperidol
Fluconazole	Meprobamate
Indomethacin	Nafcillin
L-Methyldopa	Rifampin
Metronidazole	Sucralfate
Miconazole	Tetracyclines
Omeprazole	
Phenylbutazone	
Phenytoin	
Piroxicam	
Propranolol	
Tolbutamide	
Trimethoprim-Sulfamethoxazole	

TABLE 20.5. SUGGESTED CONTRAINDICATIONS FOR THROMBOLYTIC THERAPY

Interval from onset of stroke: intravenous ≥ 4.5 hours; intra-arterial ≥ 6 hours in anterior circulation and ≥ 12 hours in posterior circulation

Rapidly resolving nondisabling neurologic signs

Treatment-refractory hypertension (inability to maintain a stable blood pressure of < 185/110 mmHg)

Diffuse swelling and hypodensity of affected hemisphere†

Computed tomographic evidence of hemorrhagic conversion

Heparin or LMWH within 48 hours

APTT > upper limit of normal

INR > 1.7

Prothrombin time < 15 seconds

Blood glucose ≤ 50 mg/dL

Platelets ≤ 100,000/mm³

Recent severe Gastrointestinal or genitourinary bleeding

Pregnancy or lactation‡

Severe traumatic brain injury within 3 months

(continued)

TABLE 20.5. (CONTINUED)

Stroke associated with infective endocarditis

Stroke due to suspected aortic arch dissection

Stroke and prior intracranial neoplasm

Stroke within past 3 months

Surgical procedure or major trauma within 14 days (consider risk in each individual case after consulting with surgeon)

---

† The size of the hypodensity is a matter of debate.

‡ With early pregnancy, may be given on a compassionate basis. Abortion may have to be granted (for more details consult the 2016 AHA/ASA scientific statement published in Stroke).

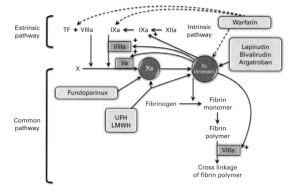

FIGURE 20.3: Mechanism of anticoagulants. UFH, unfractionated heparin; LMWH, low molecular weight heparin.

Chapter 21

Fever and Cooling

PRACTICAL NOTES

- New-onset fever often indicates infection but may be caused by resorption of blood (relative bradycardia), thromboembolism (persistent tachycardia, swollen calves), or drugs (incremental increase in temperature within several days).
- Antipyretic drugs are rarely successful and cooling devices are needed for sustained control of fever.
- Fever may prevent adequate control of seizures, intracranial pressure and delirium.
- Fever and hypotension should initiate a sepsis management protocol.

TABLE 21.1. CAUSES OF FEVER IN ACUTE NEUROLOGIC ILLNESS

Cause	Characteristics and circumstances
Nosocomial pneumonia	Pulmonary infiltrates
	Marginal oxygenation
	Ventilation-perfusion mismatch (increased alveolar-arterial gradient)
Atelectasis	Plate-like collapse of pulmonary parenchyma
Sepsis	Fever and hypotension
	Increase in leukocyte counts with shift to immature polynuclear cells
	Respiratory alkalosis (early sepsis)
Urinary tract infection	100,000 colony-forming units
	White blood cell casts
	Recent "difficult" catheterization
Decubitus ulcer infection	Preexisting spinal cord injury
	Preexisting prolonged coma

(continued)

TABLE 21.1. (CONTINUED)

Resorption of blood	Subarachnoid hemorrhage
	Traumatic brain injury
	Traumatic muscle hematomas
Thromboembolism	Persistent tachycardia
	Painful calves, calf edema, arm-hand swelling
	Increased alveolar-arterial gradient
Sinusitis	Endotracheal intubation and mechanical ventilation
Meningitis/ventriculitis	Cerebrospinal fluid leak, hematotympanum, ventriculostomy
Drug fever	New introduction (< 5 days) of drugs (e.g., penicillin, phenytoin, amphotericin B, sulfa preparations)

TABLE 21.2. FEVER EVALUATION FOR INFECTIOUS CAUSES

Fever ≥ 38.3° (≥ 101°F) for > 1 hour*

Examine access sites and catheters for inflammation or purulence

Examine surgical wounds

3–4 blood cultures within 24 hours (venipuncture rather than through device)

Chest radiograph/CT scan or consider bronchoscopy

Sputum cultures

Stool sample for C. *difficile* culture and enzyme immunoassay

Urine sample from sampling port of catheter for gram stain and microscopy

CT facial sinuses (consider aspiration or puncture sinus)

CSF (gram stain, culture, glucose, cell count), preferably from ventricular or lumbar catheter

* definition arbitrary and may be lower in elderly or immunosuppressed patients.
From O'Grady NP, Barie PS, Bartlett JG, et al. Guidelines for evaluation of new fever in critically ill adult patients: 2008 update from the American College of Critical Care Medicine and the Infectious Diseases Society of America. *Crit Care Med* 2008;36:1330–1349. With permission of the publisher.

TABLE 21.3. PROTOCOL FOR FEVER CONTROL

Fever spike	WBC, cultures, lactate
Fever spike with transient hypotension	Fluid challenge (500 mL crystalloid)
Persistent fever after spike	Cooling techniques (cooling device)
Persistent fever with persistent hypotension	Sepsis management bundle

Adapted from reference 6.

TABLE 21.4. TREATMENT OPTIONS IN SHIVERING

Intervention	Dose
Acetaminophen	650–1000 mg q 4–6 h
Buspirone	30 mg q 8 h
Magnesium sulfate	0.5–1 mg/h IV (Goal 3–4 mg/dL)
Dexmedetomidine	0.2–1.5 mcg/kg/h
Opioids	Fentanyl 100 mcg/h
	Meperidine 50–100 mg IM or IV
Propofol	50–75 mcg/kg/min
Vecuronium	0.1 mg/kg IV bolus (rarely)

Adapted from reference 6.

Chapter 22

Increased Intracranial Pressure

PRACTICAL NOTES

- Intracranial pressure must be monitored for recognition of plateau waves—sudden increases in ICP of 50–80 mm Hg lasting several minutes—which indicate failing brain compliance. Plateau waves can be muted by a change in nursing techniques and by increasing depth of sedation or intravenous administration of lidocaine or pentobarbital.
- Hypercapnia, hypoxemia, inhalation anesthetics, fever, and seizures all may increase ICP.
- The first measures to decrease ICP are head elevation to 30 degrees, treatment of agitation, and maintenance of patient comfort during mechanical ventilation.
- Traditional measures for treatment of increased ICP are CSF drainage in patients with obstructive hydrocephalus, administration of mannitol, and hyperventilation. Osmotic diuresis is the preferred first treatment. Administration of mannitol 20% is started with 1 g/kg, repeated in doses 0.5-1 g/kg aiming at a serum osmolarity of 310 mOsm/L.
- In equimolar doses hypertonic saline is equally effective as mannitol.

TABLE 22.1. CAUSES OF INCREASED
INTRACRANIAL PRESSURE

Intracranial mass
Cerebral edema
Cytotoxic (intracellular)
Vasogenic (extracellular)
Increased cerebrospinal fluid volume
Decreased absorption
Obstructed outflow
Increased production
Increased intracranial blood volume
Cerebral vasodilatation (hypoxia, hypercapnia)
Obstructed venous outflow

TABLE 22.2. DRUG EFFECTS
ON INTRACRANIAL PRESSURE

Anesthetics and sedatives	
Halothane	++
Enflurane	++
Isoflurane	++
Desflurane	++
Dexmedetomidine	±
Propofol	±
Midazolam	±
Narcotics	
Morphine	0
Alfentanil	±
Vasodilators and calcium-channel blockers	
Sodium nitroprusside	+
Hydralazine	+
Nitroglycerin	+

TABLE 22.2. (CONTINUED)

Nifedipine	+
Nicardipine	+
Nimodipine	0

++ = significant and clinically relevant; + = potentially significant; + = not clinically relevant; 0 = no change.

From Artru AA. Intracranial volume/pressure relationship during desflurane anesthesia in dogs: comparison with isoflurane and thiopental/halothane. *Anesth Analg* 1994;79:751–760; Hadley MN, Spetzler RF, Fifield MS, et al. The effect of nimodipine on intracranial pressure: volume-pressure studies in a primate model. *J Neurosurg* 1987;67:387–393; Michenfelder JD, Milde JH. The interaction of sodium nitroprusside, hypotension, and isoflurane in determining cerebral vasculature effects. *Anesthesiology* 1988;69:870–875; Papazian L, Albanese J, Thirion X, et al. Effect of bolus doses of midazolam on intracranial pressure and cerebral perfusion pressure in patients with severe head injury. *Br J Anaesth* 1993;71:267–271; Scheller MS, Todd MM, Drummond JC, et al. The intracranial pressure effects of isoflurane and halothane administered following cryogenic brain injury in rabbits. *Anesthesiology* 1987;67:507–512; Tateishi A, Sano T, Takeshita H, et al. Effects of nifedipine on intracranial pressure in neurosurgical patients with arterial hypertension. *J Neurosurg* 1988;69:213–215; Watts AD, Eliasziw M, Gelb AW. Propofol and hyperventilation for the treatment of increased intracranial pressure in rabbits. *Anesth Analg* 1998;87:564–568; Zornow MH, Scheller MS, Sheehan PB, et al. Intracranial pressure effects of dexmedetomidine in rabbits. *Anesth Analg* 1992;75:232–237. With permission of the publishers.

TABLE 22.3. OSMOLALITY
OF OSMOTIC DIURETICS COMPARED
TO NORMAL SALINE

Agent	Osmolality (mOsm/kg)
0.9% saline	308
3% saline	1026
7.5% saline	2566
23.4% saline	8008
20% mannitol	1245

TABLE 22.4. TREATMENT OF INCREASED INTRACRANIAL PRESSURE

Method	Procedure	Monitoring
Ventricular catheter	Ventricular right frontal placement with subcutaneous tunneling	CSF pressures, changes in waveform Daily calibration Drip chamber at 5–10 cm H_2O Consider prophylactic antibiotics
Hyperventilation	Increase respiratory rate to 20 breaths/min	Pco_2, 25–30 mm Hg Daily chest radiograph
Osmotic diuresis	Mannitol 20%, 1 g/kg Hypertonic saline 23%, 30 mL	Plasma osmolarity, 310–320 mOsm/L BUN, creatinine, sodium, potassium arterial blood gas, urine output
Surgical decompression	Bifrontal craniotomies Suboccipital decompression	CT scanning ICP monitor

BUN, blood urea nitrogen; CSF, cerebrospinal fluid.

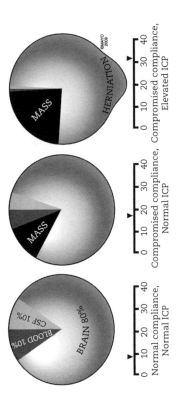

FIGURE 22.1: Illustration of compartments and compensation of increased intracranial pressure.

CSF, cerebrospinal fluid; ICP, intracranial pressure.

Part VI Technologies in the Neurosciences Intensive Care Unit

Chapter 23

Monitoring Devices

PRACTICAL NOTES

- Fiberoptic monitors are the most contemporary and reliable devices for intraparenchymal monitoring of ICP. Ventriculostomy should be reserved for patients with acute hydrocephalus.
- Continuous brain oxygen monitoring and microdialysis are research tools with the potential to become invasive monitoring devices used in daily practice. Both monitors may allow identification of brain tissue at risk.
- Jugular venous oxygen saturation may identify further insults to the brain, monitor depth of hypocapnia, and could lead to adjustment of mean arterial pressure.

TABLE 23.1. CONDITIONS THAT MAY REQUIRE MONITORING INTRACRANIAL PRESSURE

Disorder	Specific Indications
Traumatic brain injury	Any comatose patient
	Bifrontal lobe contusions and edema
	Temporal lobe contusion and edema
	Polytrauma and need for neuromuscular blockade
Aneurysmal subarachnoid hemorrhage	Acute hydrocephalus
Cerebellar stroke	Acute hydrocephalus
Encephalitis	Diffuse brain edema
Fulminant hepatic failure	Diffuse brain edema

TABLE 23.2. INDICATIONS FOR CEREBRAL OXYGENATION MONITORING

Monitoring of brain tissue exposed to ischemia
To guide hyperventilation and other measures to decrease intracranial pressure
Recognition of delayed cerebral vasospasm
Monitoring peri hematoma brain tissue exposed to mass effect

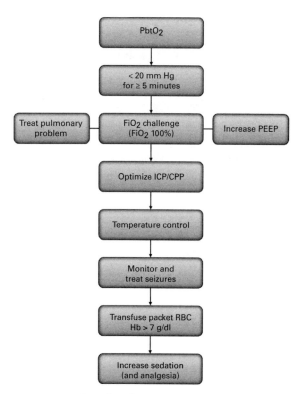

FIGURE 23.5: Clinical guide to improve cerebral oxygenation.

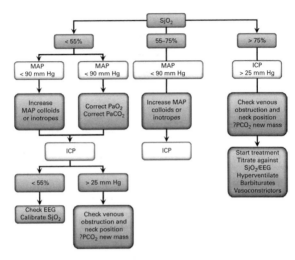

FIGURE 23.8: Guidance for interpretation of jugular bulb saturation (SjO₂). pCO2 is the partial pressure of carbon dioxide.

EEG, electroencephalogram; ICP, intracranial pressure; MAP, mean arterial pressure.

Modified from Macmillan CS, Andrews PJ. Cerebrovenous oxygen saturation monitoring: practical considerations and clinical relevance. *Intensive Care Med* 2000;26:1028–1036. With permission of Springer-Verlag.

Chapter 24

Transcranial Doppler Ultrasound and Neurophysiology

PRACTICAL NOTES

- Transcranial Doppler ultrasound is most useful in the detection of cerebral vasospasm in SAH and in the diagnosis of brain death. Typical features of cerebral vasospasm are increased mean velocities (≥120 cm/sec) and turbulence.
- Electroencephalogram is most useful in the NICU for the diagnosis of herpes simplex encephalitis, monitoring in status epilepticus, and guidance in therapy.
- Evoked potentials currently can be used only for prognostication. Poor outcome can be expected in patients with characteristic BAEP (III and IV waves absent) and SSEP (scalp potentials absent) abnormalities.
- Continuous EEG monitoring is a rapidly evolving technology with promising diagnostic capability.

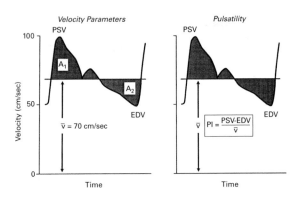

FIGURE 24.1: Typical Doppler waveform and measurement of mean velocity ($\bar{v}$) and pulsatility index (PI). *Left panel:* A cursor is placed so that the area above the cursor (A_1, defined by the peak velocity display) is equal to the area below the cursor (A_2, defined by the diastole display). *Right panel:* The PI, usually automatically calculated on transcranial Doppler machines, is the difference between the maximal and the minimal velocities, divided by the mean velocity.

EDV, end-diastolic velocity; PSV, peak systolic velocity.

Part VII Management of Specific Disorders in Critical Care Neurology

Chapter 26

Aneurysmal Subarachnoid Hemorrhage

PRACTICAL NOTES

- Basic management in SAH consists of (a) endotracheal intubation if patients cannot protect their airway, have aspirated, or have acquired neurogenic pulmonary edema; (b) adequate fluid management with 2 or 3 L of 0.9% sodium chloride; (c) no antihypertensive agents unless mean arterial pressure is more than 120 mm Hg or 160 mm Hg systolic; (d) nimodipine, 60 mg every 4 hours; and (e) pneumatic compression devices and pain management with codeine.
- The management of rebleeding consists of mechanical ventilation, antiepileptic agents if seizures occurred and emergency angiography on recovery, and early clipping or coiling.
- Delayed cerebral ischemia is managed by hemodynamic augmentation and, if this is unsuccessful, angioplasty or intra-arterial administration of verapamil or nicardipine.
- Ventriculostomy is indicated in acute hydrocephalus and hemoventricles.
- Lumbar drain placement may decrease subarachnoid blood and control ICP.

TABLE 26.1. GRADING SYSTEM
PROPOSED BY THE WORLD FEDERATION
OF NEUROLOGICAL SURGEONS FOR THE
CLASSIFICATION OF SUBARACHNOID
HEMORRHAGE

WFNS Grade	Glasgow Coma Scale Score	Motor Deficit
I	15	Absent
II	14–13	Absent
III	14–13	Present
IV	12–7	Present or absent
V	6–3	Present or absent

WFNS, World Federation of Neurological Surgeons.

TABLE 26.2. COMPUTED TOMOGRAPHY FINDINGS IN THE MODIFIED FISHER AND HIJDRA SCALE

Grade	Finding
1	Focal or diffuse thin SAH without IVH
2	Focal or diffuse thin SAH with IVH
3	Thick SAH present without IVH
4	Thick SAH present with IVH

SAH: subarachnoid hemorrhage; IVH: intraventricular hemorrhage. Data from Kistler JP, Crowell RM, Davis KR, et al. The relation of cerebral vasospasm to the extent and location of subarachnoid blood visualized by CT scan: a prospective study. *Neurology* 1983;33:424–436; and Frontera J, Claassen J, Schmidt JM, et al. Prediction of symptomatic vasospasm after subarachnoid hemorrhage: the modified Fisher scale. *Neurosurgery* 2006;59:21–27.

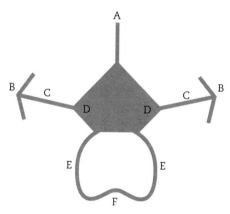

Hijdra method of grading subarachnoid hemorrhage identifies 10 basal cisterns and fissures: (A) frontal interhemispheric fissure; (B) sylvian fissure, lateral parts both sides; (C) sylvian fissure, basal parts both sides; (D) suprasellar cistern both sides; (E) ambient cisterns both sides; and (F) quadrigeminal cistern. The amount of blood in each cistern and fissure is graded 0, no blood; 1, small amount of blood; 2, moderately filled with blood; and 3, completely filled with blood. The sum score is 0 to 30 points.

TABLE 26.3. INITIAL MANAGEMENT OF ANEURYSMAL SUBARACHNOID HEMORRHAGE

Airway management	Intubation if patient has hypoxemia despite facemask with 10 L of 60%–100% oxygen/minute, if abnormal respiratory drive or if abnormal protective reflexes (likely with motor response of withdrawal or worse)
Mechanical ventilation	IMV/PS AC with aspiration pneumonitis, ARDS or early neurogenic pulmonary edema
Fluid management	2–3 L of 0.9% NaCl per 24 hours Fludrocortisone acetate, 0.2 mg b.i.d. orally, if patient has hyponatremia
Blood pressure management	Aim at SBP of < 160 mm Hg IV labetalol 10–15 mg every 15 min if needed Hydralazine 10–20 mg IV if bradycardia
Nutrition	Enteral nutrition with continuous infusion (on day 2) Blood glucose control (goal 140–180 mg/dL)
Prophylaxis	DVT prophylaxis with pneumatic compression devices SC heparin 5,000 U t.i.d. after clipping or coiling of aneurysm GI prophylaxis: pantoprazole 40 mg IV daily or lansoprazole 30 mg orally through nasogastric tube.

Other measures	Nimodipine, 60 mg six times a day orally for 21 days
	Tranexamic acid 1 gram IV, second dose 2 hours later, third dose 6 hours later if delayed clipping or coiling
	Codeine 30–60 mg orally every 4 hours as needed
	Tramadol, 50–100 mg orally q4h, for pain management
	Levetiracetam 20 mg/kg IV over 60 minutes; 1,000 mg b.i.d. maintenance (if seizures have occurred)
Access	Arterial catheter to monitor blood pressure (if IV antihypertensive drugs anticipated)
	Peripheral venous catheter or peripheral inserted central catheter

ARDS, acute respiratory distress syndrome; DVT, deep vein thrombosis; GI, gastrointestinal; IMV, intermittent mandatory ventilation; IV, intravenously; MAP, mean arterial pressure; NaCl, sodium chloride; PS, pressure support; SBP, systolic blood pressure; SC, subcutaneously.

TABLE 26.4. PROTOCOL FOR EUVOLEMIC HYPERTENSION IN THE TREATMENT OF CEREBRAL VASOSPASM IN ANEURYSMAL SUBARACHNOID HEMORRHAGE

SAH, clinically asymptomatic but TCD or CT (angiogram or perfusion) evidence of diffuse cerebral vasospasm

Obtain hourly readings of fluid balance and body weight

Accomplish volume repletion with crystalloids

Avoid antihypertensive and diuretic agents

SAH, secured aneurysm, clinical evidence of cerebral vasospasm

Notify neurointerventionalist for possible cerebral angiography

Give crystalloid bolus or albumin 5%

Match fluid input with urine output

When urine output is > 250 mL/hr, start administration of fludrocortisone acetate, 0.2 mg b.i.d.

Concurrently start administration of IV phenylephrine, 10–30 μg/min, with increase in MAP 25% above baseline or > 120 mm Hg (a central access is secured).

Start administration of IV dobutamine, 5–15 μg/kg/min if no response.

Consider replacing phenylephrine with norepinephrine if no response.

Perform cerebral angiography for angioplasty or intra-arterial infusion with verapamil.

CT, computed tomography; MAP, mean arterial pressure; SAH, subarachnoid hemorrhage; TCD, transcranial Doppler ultrasonography.

TABLE 26.5. COMMONLY USED HEMODYNAMIC AGENTS
IN SUBARACHNOID HEMORRHAGE

Agent	Action	Dose	Side Effect
Dobutamine	β_1 agonist ($\uparrow$CO) β_2 stimulation ($\downarrow$SVR)	5–40 µg/kg/min	Tachycardia (often when hypovolemic)
Dopamine	Low dose (0.5–3 µg/kg/min) →renal vasodilatation →small decrease in BP High dose (10–20 µg/kg/min) ($\uparrow\beta_2$ receptors) $\uparrow$increase in CO $\uparrow$increase in BP	1–20 µg/kg/min	Tachyarrhythmia (common)
Phenylephrine	agonist ($\uparrow$SVR) No effect on CO	10–30 µg/min	Reflex bradycardia

BP, blood pressure; CO, cardiac output; SVR, systemic vascular resistance. (Also see appendix for titration schedule.)

TABLE 26.6. INTRA-ARTERIAL AGENTS
TO IMPROVE CEREBRAL VASOSPASM

Agent	t1/2	Improvement Arteries vs. Clinical
Papaverine[85]	2 hours	43% vs. n/a
Verapamil[52]	7 hours	44% vs. 33%
Nicardipine[4,150]	16 hours	60% vs. 91%
Nimodipine[9]	9 hours	43% vs. 76%

n/a = not available.

TABLE 26.7. CONTRAINDICATIONS FOR LUMBAR DRAIN PLACEMENT IN ANEURYSMAL SUBARACHNOID HEMORRHAGE

Any hemispheric or extracranial hematoma with mass effect or shift of midline structures

Effacement of the basilar cisterns

Obstructive clot in third or fourth ventricle

Coagulopathy (INR > 1.4)

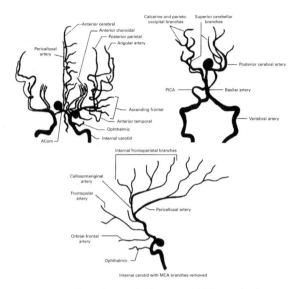

FIGURE 26.6: Anterior cerebral artery, middle cerebral artery, basilar artery tip, and posterior communicating artery aneurysms on cerebral angiogram in their optimal projections.

ACom, anterior communicating artery; MCA, middle cerebral artery; PICA, posterior inferior cerebellar artery.

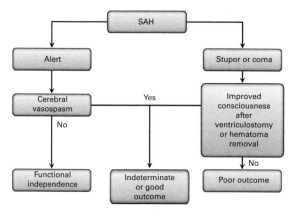

FIGURE 26.15: Outcome algorithm. Functional independence: No assistance needed, minor handicap may remain. Indeterminate: Any statement would be a premature conclusion. Poor outcome: Severe disability, persistent vegetative state, or death.

SAH, subarachnoid hemorrhage.

Chapter 27

Ganglionic and Lobar Hemorrhages

PRACTICAL NOTES

- Medical management includes correction of possible coagulopathy (preferred Prothrombin complex concentrate and vitamin K, but can consider factor VIIa and fresh frozen plasma), control of mass effect and shift (3% hypertonic saline or mannitol, 1 g/kg), early control of blood pressure to 160 mmHg with IV antihypertensives and antiepileptic drugs for 2–3 weeks in lobar hematoma only.
- Neurosurgical intervention is considered for marked clinical deterioration but outcome in treated patients with ganglionic hemorrhages is not much better. Early surgical intervention is indicated in superficially located hematoma and brain tissue shift.

TABLE 27.1. GRAEBE SCALE: SYSTEM FOR GRADING SEVERITY OF IVH

Lateral Ventricles

1 = trace of blood or mild bleeding

2 = less than half of the ventricle filled with blood

3 = more than half of the ventricle filled with blood

4 = ventricle filled with blood and expanded

(Each lateral ventricle is scored separately)

Third and Fourth Ventricles

1 = blood present, ventricle size normal

2 = ventricle filled with blood and expanded

Total Score (maximum = 12)

TABLE 27.2. LABORATORY TESTS IN CEREBRAL HEMORRHAGE

Complete white cell count, platelet count, blood smear, sedimentation rate

Activated partial thromboplastin time, international normalized ratio

Aspartate transaminase, alkaline phosphatase

Fibrinogen and fibrinogen split products (optional)

Transthoracic echocardiography and serial blood cultures (optional)

Human immunodeficiency virus serology (optional)

Drug screen (optional)

Hemoglobin electrophoresis (optional)

TABLE 27.3. INITIAL MANAGEMENT OF GANGLIONIC AND LOBAR HEMORRHAGES

Airway management	Intubation if patient has hypoxemia despite facemask with 10 L of 60%–100% oxygen/minute, if abnormal respiratory drive or if abnormal protective reflexes (likely with motor response of withdrawal, or worse)
Mechanical ventilation	IMV/PS
	AC with aspiration pneumonitis
	Increase IMV to 15 when hyperventilation is indicated
Fluid management	2–3 L of 0.9% NaCl
	Mannitol, 1 g/kg, when shift appears on CT scan and patient deteriorates rapidly
Blood pressure management	Aim at systolic blood pressure between 130–140 mm Hg. IV labetalol, 10–15 mg every 15 min if needed. Hydralazine 10–20 mg IV if bradycardia. Consider nicardipine 5 mg/hr IV (maximum 15 mg/hr IV)
Nutrition	Enteral nutrition with continuous infusion (on day 2)
	Blood glucose control (goal 140–180 mg/dL)

Prophylaxis	DVT prophylaxis with pneumatic devices
	SC heparin 5,000 U t.i.d. after surgical evacuation or 2 days after ictus
	GI prophylaxis: pantoprazole 40 mg IV daily or lansoprazole 30 mg orally through nasogastric tube
	Levetiracetam 20 mg/kg IV over 60 minutes followed by 1,000 mg b.i.d. maintenance in lobar hematoma only
Other measures	Reverse anticoagulation (Table 27.4)
Surgical management	Evacuate hematoma if patient is deteriorating and has a lobar hematoma with shift
Access	Arterial catheter to monitor blood pressure (if IV antihypertensive drugs anticipated)
	Peripheral venous catheter or peripheral inserted central catheter

CT, computed tomography; DVT, deep vein thrombosis; GI, gastrointestinal; IMV, intermittent mandatory ventilation; IV, intravenously; MAP, mean arterial pressure; NaCl, sodium chloride; PS, pressure support; SC, subcutaneously.

TABLE 27.4. ANTICOAGULATION
REVERSAL

Warfarin

Fresh frozen plasma (2 Units), vitamin K, 10 mg IV

Factor VIIa 10–20 mcg/kg in one infusion

PCC 30–50 IU/kg.

Heparin

Stop infusion

Protamine sulfate, 1 mg per 100 U of heparin
(maximal dose 50 mg)

Low molecular weight heparin

If within 12 hours, 1 mg protamine for each 1 mg of
enoxaparin

Protamine not useful in LMWH when administered
after 12 hours

Protamine does not reverse fondaparinux

IV tPA

Stop infusion

Tranexamic acid 1 gram in 20 minutes

Cryoprecipitate (0.15 U/kg) if fibrinogen is < 150
mg/dL

Platelet transfusion if platelets < 100 × 109/L

Thrombin inhibitors

Oral activated charcoal (if within 2 hours ingestion)

PCC 50 IU/kg

Hemodialysis (dabigatran only)

Monoclonal antibodies

Antiplatelets

Consider 2 units of platelets when prior use of dual
antiplatelet therapy and surgery is anticipated.

TABLE 27.5. SPETZLER-MARTIN GRADING SYSTEM FOR ARTERIOVENOUS MALFORMATIONS

Variable	Score*
Size of arteriovenous malformation†	
Small (< 3 cm)	1
Medium (3–6 cm)	2
Large (> 6 cm)	3
Eloquence of adjacent brain‡	
No	0
Yes	1
Patterns of venous drainage§	
Superficial only	0
Deep	1

* Score of 1 equals grade I, score of 2 equals grade II, etc.
† Greatest diameter on magnetic resonance imaging, cerebral angiography, or computed tomography scan.
‡ Eloquent or functionally important areas are sensory-motor, language, visual cortex, diencephalon, internal capsule, brainstem, and peduncles or deep nuclei of the cerebellum.
§ Deep venous drainage and deep perforating arterial feeders.
From Martin NA, Vinters HV. Arteriovenous malformations. In Carter LP, Spetzler RF, eds., *Neurovascular Surgery.* New York: McGraw-Hill, 1995:875–903. With permission of the publisher.

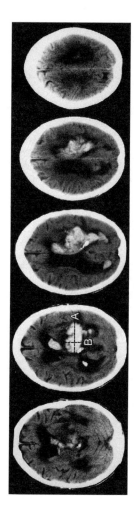

FIGURE 27.1: Volume of a thalamic hemorrhage as measured by the ABC method (A × B × C). In this example, A is 5 cm, B is 3 cm, and the number of slices (C) is four (hemorrhage is visible on four computed tomographic slices at 1 cm intervals). The total volume is calculated as 60 divided by 2, or 30 cm3.

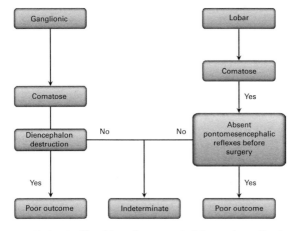

FIGURE 27.15: Algorithm of outcome in lobar and ganglionic intracranial hemorrhages.

Poor outcome: Severe disability or death, vegetative state.

Indeterminate: Any statement would be a premature conclusion.

Chapter 28

Cerebellum and Brainstem Hemorrhages

PRACTICAL NOTES

- The CT scan signs in cerebellar hemorrhages are disappearance of the fourth ventricle, compression of ambient and quadrigeminal cisterns, and squaring off of the peritectal cistern, features most often seen in hematomas larger than 3 cm.
- Suboccipital decompressive craniotomy is the mainstay of management for large cerebellar hematomas.
- Management of cerebellar hematoma includes elective intubation in patients with rapid impairment of consciousness, mannitol in patients with CT evidence of tight posterior fossa, and labetalol intravenously for blood pressure control. Runs of bradycardia can be treated with atropine.
- Suboccipital craniotomy in comatose patients with cerebellar hemorrhage and loss of some brainstem reflexes may still result in independent recovery, but this is less likely when corneal reflexes are absent.
- Primary pontine hemorrhages carry a high mortality, often in patients with hyperthermia at presentation, intraventricular hematoma, and extension to midbrain and thalamus.
- In patients with a small localized hemorrhage, MRI studies are needed to demonstrate a possible arteriovenous malformation that can be successfully removed surgically.

TABLE 28.1. INITIAL MANAGEMENT OF CEREBELLAR HEMATOMA

Airway management	Intubation if patient has hypoxemia despite facemask with 10 L of 60%–100% oxygen/minute, if abnormal respiratory drive or if abnormal protective reflexes (likely with motor response of withdrawal, or worse)
Mechanical ventilation	IMV/PS or CPAP mode
Fluid management	2–3 L of 0.9% NaCl
	Mannitol, 1 g/kg bolus, in patients with tight posterior fossa on CT scans. May consider 3%–23% hypertonic saline if a central access is available or pushing it through a femoral vein.
Blood pressure management	Labetalol, 10–20 mg IV every 15 min if needed for persistent hypertension (MAP > 130 mm Hg); hydralazine 10–20 mg IV if bradycardia
Cardiac arrhythmias	Sinus bradycardia: atropine, 0.5–2.0 mg IV
	Sinus tachycardia: fluid bolus, 500 mL of 0.9% NaCl or 250 mL of albumin 5%; metoprolol 5 mg IV
Nutrition	Enteral nutrition with continuous infusion (on day 2)
	Blood glucose control (goal 140–180 mg/dL)

(continued)

TABLE 28.1. (CONTINUED)

Prophylaxis	DVT prophylaxis with pneumatic compression devices
	SC heparin 5000 U t.i.d. 2 days after craniotomy
	GI prophylaxis: pantoprazole 40 mg IV daily or lansoprazole 30 mg orally through nasogastric tube.
Surgical management	Surgical evacuation: hematoma size > 3 cm, obliterated 4th ventricle, or collapsed quadrigeminal cistern on CT scan
	Ventriculostomy for acute hydrocephalus
Access	Arterial catheter to monitor blood pressure (if IV antihypertensive drugs anticipated)
	Peripheral venous catheter or peripheral inserted central catheter

CPAP, continuous positive airway pressure; CT, computed tomography; DVT, deep vein thrombosis; GI, gastrointestinal; IMV, intermittent mandatory ventilation; IV, intravenously; MAP, mean arterial pressure; NaCl, sodium chloride; PS, pressure support; SC, subcutaneously.

TABLE 28.2. INITIAL MANAGEMENT OF BRAINSTEM HEMORRHAGE

Airway management	Intubation if patient has hypoxemia despite facemask with 10 L of 100% oxygen/minute, if abnormal respiratory drive or if abnormal protective reflexes (likely with abnormal motor response of withdrawal, or worse)
Mechanical ventilation	IMV/PS or CPAP mode
Fluid management	2–3 L of 0.9% NaCl; increase amount in hyperthermia to 1 L per 1°C increase in temperature
Blood pressure management	Labetalol, 10–20 mg IV every 15 min if needed, for persistent hypertension (MAP > 120 mm Hg); hydralazine 10–20 mg IV if bradycardia.
Nutrition	Enteral nutrition with continuous infusion (on day 2)
	Blood glucose control (goal 140–180 mg/dL).
Prophylaxis	DVT prophylaxis with pneumatic compression devices
	GI prophylaxis: pantoprazole 40 mg IV daily or lansoprazole 30 mg orally through nasogastric tube
Access	Arterial catheter to monitor blood pressure (if IV antihypertensive drugs anticipated);
	peripheral venous catheter or peripheral inserted central catheter

CPAP, continuous positive airway pressure; DVT, deep vein thrombosis; GI, gastrointestinal; IMV, intermittent mandatory ventilation; IV, intravenously; MAP, mean arterial pressure; NaCl, sodium chloride; PS, pressure support.

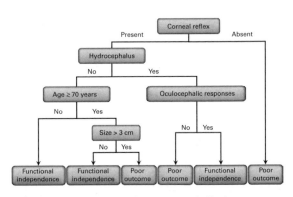

FIGURE 28.6: Outcome predictors in cerebellar hematoma.

Poor outcome: Severe disability or death, vegetative state. Functional independence: No assistance needed, minor handicap may remain.

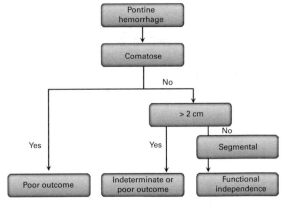

FIGURE 28.7: Outcome predictors in primary pontine hemorrhage.

Poor outcome: Severe disability or death, vegetative state.

Indeterminate: Any statement would be a premature conclusion.

Functional independence: No assistance needed, minor handicap may remain.

Chapter 29

Major Hemispheric Ischemic Stroke Syndromes

PRACTICAL NOTES

- The anatomy of vascular occlusion may indicate certain cause and direction of intervention.
- Acute occlusive disease can be treated with IV and IA thrombolytics, mechanical disruption, or stenting, and all three options can be considered.
- Deterioration in patients with MCA occlusion consists of brain swelling, cerebral hematoma from hemorrhagic conversion, or pulmonary edema due to aspiration or fluid overload.
- Primary control of brain swelling may initially with scheduled mannitol or hypertonic saline. Decompressive surgery or hypothermia should be considered.

TABLE 29.2. INITIAL MANAGEMENT OF ACUTE HEMISPHERIC INFARCTION

Airway management	Intubation if patient has hypoxemia despite facemask with 10 L of 100% oxygen/minute, if abnormal respiratory drive or if abnormal protective reflexes (likely with motor response of withdrawal, or worse)
Mechanical ventilation	IMV/PS or CPAP mode
Fluid management	2–3 L of 0.9% NaCl per 24 hours
	Rehydrate with 500 mL of normal saline or albumin 5%
Blood pressure management	No antihypertensive agents unless MAP > 120 mm Hg
Nutrition	Enteral nutrition with continuous infusion (on day 2)
	Blood glucose control (goal 140–180 mg/dL)
Prophylaxis	DVT prophylaxis with pneumatic compression devices
	SC heparin 5,000 U t.i.d.
	GI prophylaxis: pantoprazole 40 mg IV daily or lansoprazole 30 mg orally through nasogastric tube
Other measures	Maintain normothermia with cooling blankets
Access	Arterial catheter to monitor blood pressure (if IV antihypertensive drugs anticipated)
	Peripheral venous catheter or peripheral inserted central catheter

CPAP, continuous positive airway pressure; DVT, deep vein thrombosis; GI, gastrointestinal; IMV, intermittent mandatory ventilation; IV, intravenously; MAP, mean arterial pressure; NaCl, sodium chloride; PS, pressure support; SC, subcutaneously.

TABLE 29.3. TREATMENT OPTIONS
FOR CEREBRAL SWELLING
IN HEMISPHERIC INFARCTION

Maintain adequate hydration but restrict free water

Assess the effect of mannitol 20%, 1 g/kg

If mannitol is unsuccessful, place central catheter
and administer repeated doses of 30 mL of 23%
saline

If hypertonic saline therapy is unsuccessful, consider
decompressive hemicraniectomy

If decompressive hemicraniectomy is refused or
unsuccessful, consider hypothermia therapy,
reducing core body temperature to 33°–34°C by
using cooling blankets or cooling devices, gastric
lavage with ice water, and alcohol rubbing

Treat shivering with propofol (up to 3–5 mcg/kg/hr)
and alfentanil (0.5–3 µg/kg/min) if needed

Monitor serum amylase, activated partial
thromboplastin time, platelet count, and troponin
daily during hypothermia

Continue hypothermia for 3 days and rewarm,
ideally increasing temperature 1°C every 6 hours

CAPSULE 29.1   DECOMPRESSIVE HEMICRANIECTOMY AND OUTCOME

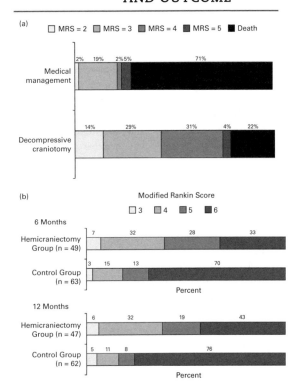

(a) Outcome in pooled analysis of hemicraniectomy trials. Outcomes are assessed with modified Rankin Scale (mRS). Poor outcome is generally considered mRS 3 or more.
(b) Outcome of decompressive surgery in elderly.

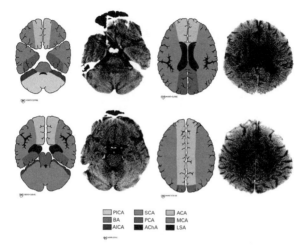

	PICA		SCA		ACA
	BA		PCA		MCA
	AICA		AChA		LSA

FIGURE 29.2: Vascular territories of the brain (computed tomographic scans and corresponding arterial territories).

ACA, anterior cerebral artery; AChA, anterior choroidal artery; AICA, anterior inferior cerebellar artery; BA, basilar artery; LSA, lenticulostriate artery; MCA, middle cerebral artery; PCA, posterior cerebral artery; PICA, posterior inferior cerebellar artery; SCA, superior cerebellar artery.

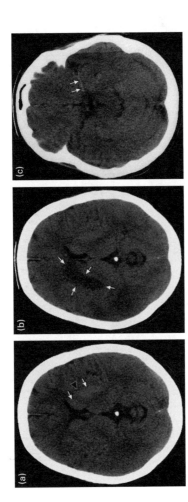

FIGURE 29.3. (a) Normal definition of the caudate nucleus, lentiform nucleus (*arrows*), and insular ribbon (*arrowhead*) in the left hemisphere has disappeared in the right hemisphere. (b) One day later, a computed tomography (CT) scan shows a hypodensity in that area (c) Hyperdense middle cerebral artery sign (*arrows*).

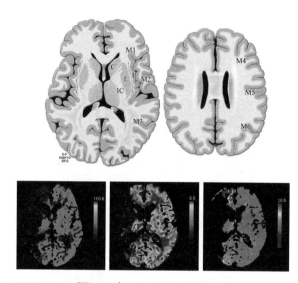

FIGURE 29.7: CT scan showing ASPECTS (0–10) one point subtracted for ischemic change in each region. Reconsideration thrombolytic or endovascular treatment with ASPECT of 6 or less. Perfusion CT scans in acute MCA stroke. From left to right note match between the cerebral blood flow, cerebral blood volume and time to peak.

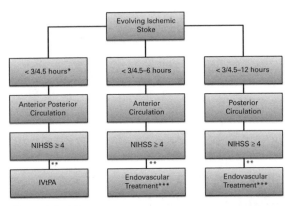

*No contraindications
***May be MRI/DWI or CTA/P guided

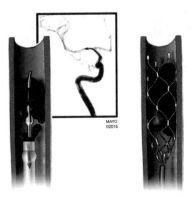

FIGURE 29.14: Decisions in acute evolving ischemic stroke. Endovascular treatment is now with stent retrievers or suction/aspiration devices.

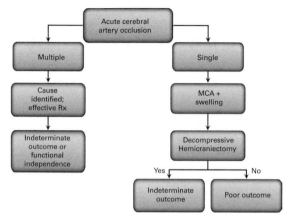

FIGURE 29.19: Outcome algorithm in hemispheric strokes. Poor outcome: Severe disability or death, vegetative state. Indeterminate: Any statement would be a premature conclusion. Functional independence or good outcome: No assistance needed, minor handicap may remain.

Chapter 30

Acute Basilar Artery Occlusion

PRACTICAL NOTES

- Tissue plasminogen activator, 90 mg intravenous dose in 1 hour (10% in bolus, 90% by infusion), should be considered standard before endovascular treatment.
- Endovascular treatment should be considered in patients with acute basilar artery occlusion seen within 12 hours.
- Standard management includes heparin (aPTT 1.5–2 times the control value). In patients with hypotension, consider further blood pressure support with flat body position and phenylephrine to achieve a mean arterial pressure 110–130 mm Hg.
- Mechanical ventilation for apneic episodes, persistent coma for 1 week, and MRI showing entire pontine infarction carry a very poor prognosis.
- Good outcome can be expected in patients with a slowly progressive clinical course, limited neurologic deficits, short segmental abnormalities, and good collateral flow on cerebral angiography.

TABLE 30.1. INITIAL MANAGEMENT OF ACUTE BASILAR ARTERY OCCLUSION

Airway management	Intubation if patient has hypoxemia despite facemask with 10 L of 60%–100% oxygen/minute, if abnormal respiratory drive or if abnormal protective reflexes (likely with motor response of withdrawal, or worse)
Mechanical ventilation	IMV/PS or CPAP mode; AC with aspiration pneumonitis
Fluid management	Maintenance with 3 L of 0.9% NaCl: Flat body position
Blood pressure management	Blood pressure augmentation with IV phenylephrine to mean arterial pressure of 100–120 mm Hg can be considered
Nutrition	Enteral nutrition with continuous infusion (on day 2)
	Blood glucose control (goal 140–180 mg/dL)
Prophylaxis	DVT prophylaxis with pneumatic compression devices
	SC heparin 5000 U t.i.d.
	GI prophylaxis: pantoprazole 40 mg IV daily or lansoprazole 30 mg orally through nasogastric tube.
Endovascular therapy	Mechanical retrieval of clot and possibly angioplasty
	Intraarterial tissue plasminogen activator
Access	Arterial catheter to monitor blood pressure (if vasopressors are anticipated)
	Peripheral venous catheter or Peripheral inserted central catheter

AC, Assist control; CPAP, continuous positive airway pressure; DVT, deep vein thrombosis; GI, gastrointestinal; IMV, intermittent mandatory ventilation; IV, intravenously; NaCl, sodium chloride; PS, pressure support; SC, subcutaneously.

CAPSULE 30.1   THE CLASSIC BRAINSTEM SYNDROMES

Eponym	Lesion	Features
Midbrain		
Weber	Cerebral peduncle	Ipsilateral III nerve palsy
		Contralateral hemiparesis
Benedikt	Tegmentum, red nucleus	Ipsilateral III nerve palsy
		Contralateral tremor, chorea
Parinaud	Quadrigeminal plate	Paralysis of upward gaze
Chiray-Foix-Nicolesco	Lateral mesencephalon	Hemiataxia
		Hemichorea
		Decreased vibration and proprioception
		Arm and leg weakness with or without facial weakness

Pons		
Raymond	Paramedian area	Ipsilateral lateral rectus muscle paresis, contralateral hemiplegia
Millard-Gubler	Medial lower	Ipsilateral facial palsy with contralateral hemiplegia (often also VI)
Foville	Medial lower	Ipsilateral VII Ipsilateral paralysis of lateral gaze Contralateral hemiparesis
Raymond-Céstan	Medial	Quadriplegia Anesthesia Nystagmus
Brissaud	Ventral	Ipsilateral facial spasm Contralateral hemiparesis

(continued)

CAPSULE 30.1   (CONTINUED)

Eponym	Lesion	Features
Medulla Oblongata		
Wallenberg	Lateral	Horner's syndrome (ipsilateral), IX, X
		Crossed hemianesthesia
Avellis	Nucleus ambiguus	X, XI palsy (ipsilateral face, contralateral body)
	Spinothalamic tract	Tractus solitarius
		Contralateral dissociated hemianesthesia
Schmidt	Vagal nuclei	X, XI
	Bulbar and spinal nuclei of accessory fibers	
Jackson	Nuclear vagus, accessory, Hypoglossus nerve	X, XI, XII
Tapia	Motor nuclei vagus and Hypoglossus	X, XII

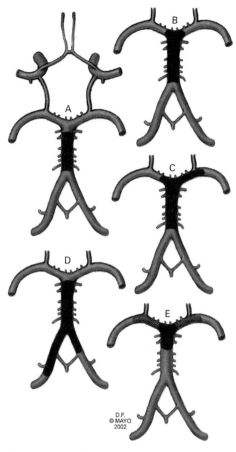

FIGURE 30.1: Sites of basilar artery occlusion.
Most likely as deduced from clinicopathologic correlation, (A) a
thrombus occludes the paramedian or short circumferential
branch, with possible further extension into the basilar artery
(B), posterior cerebral artery (C), or vertebral artery (D). An
embolus or thrombus may also lodge at the tip of the basilar
artery (E), occluding supply to the thalamus, cerebral peduncle,
and temporal and occipital lobes.

Modified from Kubik CS, Adams RD. Occlusion of the basilar artery: a
clinical and pathological study. *Brain* 1946;69:73–121. With permission
of Oxford University Press.

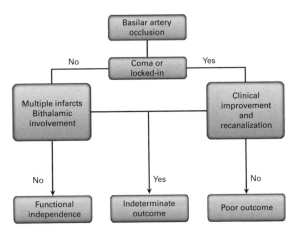

FIGURE 30.8: Outcome algorithm in acute basilar artery occlusion.

Functional independence: No assistance needed, minor handicap may remain. Indeterminate: Any statement would be a premature conclusion. Poor outcome: Severe disability, prolonged comatose state, or death.

Chapter 31

Cerebellar Infarct

PRACTICAL NOTES

- Important CT scan criteria for the diagnosis of cerebellar swelling are hypodensity with obliteration of the fourth ventricle, brainstem deformity, obstructive hydrocephalus, and obliteration of the ambient cistern. Magnetic resonance imaging findings of brainstem displacement do not predict deterioration.
- Patients with PICA infarcts have a 30% risk of further deterioration from swelling.
- Symptoms of brainstem compression are gaze deviation in the horizontal plane, disappearing corneal reflexes, paralysis of upward gaze, and pinpoint pupils.
- Definitive management of cerebellar infarcts remains suboccipital craniotomy in patients with deterioration or who fail to improve. Ventriculostomy is considered only if deterioration is from obstructive hydrocephalus alone.

TABLE 31.1. CLINICAL SYNDROMES OF INFARCTION IN THE DISTRIBUTION OF THE CEREBELLAR ARTERIES

Arterial Territory	Structures Affected	Clinical Manifestations
Posterior inferior cerebellar artery	Restiform body, inferior surface of cerebellar hemisphere	Limb ataxia, gait ataxia
	Descending tract and nucleus of fifth nerve	Facial hypesthesia to pain and temperature
	Nucleus ambiguus	Palatal weakness, decreased gag reflex, dystonia (vocal cord paresis)
	Descending sympathetic tract	Horner's syndrome
	Spinothalamic tract	Hypesthesia to pain and temperature of limbs and trunk
	Vestibular nuclei	Vertigo, nystagmus
Anterior inferior cerebellar artery	Brachium pontis, inferior surface of cerebellar hemisphere	Limb ataxia, gait ataxia
	Descending sympathetic tract	Horner syndrome
	Cochlear nucleus	Deafness
		Facial paralysis

	Intrapontine course of seventh nerve	Facial hypesthesia
	Trigeminal nuclei (descending tract and main sensory tract)	Hypesthesia to pain and temperature of limbs and trunk
	Spinothalamic tract	Vertigo, nystagmus
	Vestibular nuclei	
Superior cerebellar artery	Brachium pontis, superior surface of cerebellar hemisphere (including vermis), dentate nucleus	Limb ataxia, gait ataxia
	Brachium conjunctivum	Choreiform dyskinesia
	Descending sympathetic tract	Horner's syndrome
	Spinothalamic tract	Hypesthesia to pain and temperature of limbs and trunk
	Pontine tectum	Trochlear nerve palsy

Modified from Kase CS. Cerebellar infarction. *Heart Dis Stroke* 1994;3:38–45. With permission of the American Heart Association.

TABLE 31.2. INITIAL MANAGEMENT OF CEREBELLAR INFARCT

Airway management	Intubation if patient has hypoxemia despite face mask of 10% oxygen/min, if abnormal respiratory drive or if abnormal protective reflexes, likely with motor response of withdrawal or worse
Mechanical ventilation	IMV/PS or CPAP mode
Fluid management	2 L of 0.9% NaCl
Blood pressure management	No treatment of hypertension unless persistently MAP > 130 mm Hg
Nutrition	Assess swallowing mechanism and place nasogastric tube
	Enteral nutrition with continuous infusion (on day 2)
	Blood glucose control (goal 140–180 mg/dL)
Prophylaxis	DVT prophylaxis with pneumatic compression devices
	Consider SC heparin 5000 U t.i.d.
	GI prophylaxis: pantoprazole 40 mg IV daily or lansoprazole 30 mg orally through nasogastric tube
Other measures	Heparin IV (activated partial thromboplastin time twice control value)
	Baclofen for hiccups (15 mg qid orally)

Surgical Management	Ventriculostomy if progressive hydrocephalus but no compression of the brainstem
	Suboccipital decompressive craniotomy if further neurologic deterioration from brainstem compression
Access	Arterial catheter to monitor blood pressure (if IV antihypertensive drugs anticipated)
	Peripheral venous catheter or peripheral inserted central catheter

CPAP, continuous positive airway pressure; DVT, deep vein thrombosis; GI, gastrointestinal; IMV, intermittent mandatory ventilation; IV, intravenously; MAP, mean arterial pressure; NaCl, sodium chloride; PS, pressure support; SC, subcutaneously.

CAPSULE 31.1 VASCULARIZATION OF THE CEREBELLUM

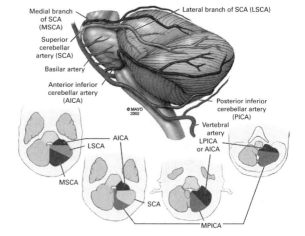

Vascular bed of cerebellum. Serial horizontal cuts identify single territories.

LPICA, lateral branch of posterior inferior cerebellar artery; MPICA, medial branch of posterior inferior cerebellar artery.

Modified from Amarenco P. The spectrum of cerebellar infarctions. *Neurology* 1991;41:973–979.

With permission of the American Academy of Neurology.

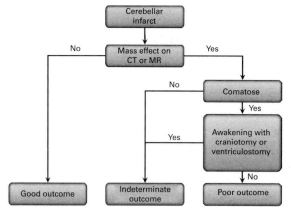

FIGURE 31.4: Outcome algorithm for cerebellar infarction. Good outcome: No assistance needed, minor handicap may remain. Indeterminate outcome: Any statement would be a premature conclusion. Poor outcome: Severe disability or death, vegetative state.

CT, computed tomography; MR, magnetic resonance imaging.

Chapter 32

Cerebral Venous Thrombosis

PRACTICAL NOTES

- Magnetic resonance imaging and gadolinium bolus MRV remain the preferred diagnostic tests. Cerebral angiography should be performed if thrombolysis is considered.
- Management consists of rehydration, rapid anticoagulation with heparin to an activated partial thromboplastin time of two times the control value, and control of intracranial pressure in comatose patients.
- Intravenous administration of heparin should be continued in patients with hemorrhagic infarcts or hematomas without mass effect.
- Increased intracranial pressure can be controlled by hyperventilation (diffuse edema or bilateral cerebral infarcts), or barbiturates.
- Evacuation of a hemorrhagic infarct may be needed in deteriorating patients from mass effect.

TABLE 32.1. LABORATORY STUDIES IN PATIENTS WITH CEREBRAL VENOUS THROMBOSIS

Blood smear, platelet count, differential count

Antithrombin III, protein C, and protein S

Heparin cofactor II

Plasma fibrinogen

Lupus anticoagulant

Anticardiolipin antibodies

MTHFR mutation

Plasma homocysteine

Hemoglobin electrophoresis

Urinalysis with quantification of protein and determination of hemosiderin

Coombs test, rheumatoid factor, antineutrophil cytoplasmic autoantibody, antinuclear antibody

Drug screen

Computed tomography scan of chest or abdomen, or both

Optional

    Human immunodeficiency virus

    Colonoscopy

    Skin and conjunctiva biopsy

    Blood cultures

    Bone marrow

    Hematology consultation

    Rheumatology consultation

    Otorhinolaryngology consultation

MTHFR, methylenetetrahydrofolate reductase.

TABLE 32.2. INITIAL MANAGEMENT OF CEREBRAL VENOUS THROMBOSIS

Airway management	Intubation if patient has hypoxemia despite face mask with 10 L of 100% oxygen/minute, if abnormal respiratory drive or presence of abnormal protective reflexes (likely with motor response of withdrawal, or worse)
Mechanical ventilation	IMV/PS or CPAP in most patients
Fluid management	Rapid hydration with normal saline
	Maintenance fluid intake, 3 L of 0.9% NaCl
Nutrition	Enteral nutrition with continuous infusion (on day 2)
	Blood glucose control (goal 140–180 mg/dL)
Prophylaxis	DVT prophylaxis with pneumatic compression devices
	GI prophylaxis: pantoprazole 40 mg IV daily or lansoprazole 30 mg orally through nasogastric tube.
Other measures	Heparin infusion, per weight based nomogram, activated partial thromboplastin time two times control
	Endovascular thrombolysis
	Fenestration can be considered if papilledema is present
Access	Peripheral venous catheter or peripheral inserted central catheter

CPAP, continuous positive airway pressure; DVT, deep vein thrombosis; GI, gastrointestinal; IMV, intermittent mandatory ventilation; IV, intravenously; NaCl, sodium chloride; PS, pressure support.

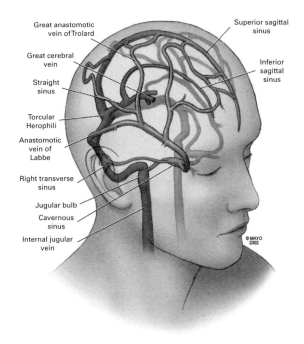

FIGURE 32.1: Anatomy of the cerebral venous system. The superficial and deep draining veins are depicted with anastomoses.

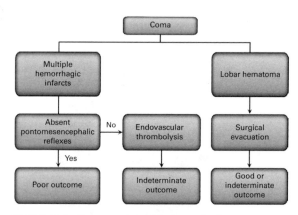

FIGURE 32.8: Outcome algorithm for cerebral venous thrombosis. Functional independence: No assistance needed, minor handicap may remain. Poor outcome: Severe disability or death, vegetative state. Indeterminate: Any statement would be a premature conclusion.

Chapter 33

Acute Bacterial Meningitis

PRACTICAL NOTES

- *S. pneumoniae* is the cause of most cases of adult bacterial meningitis. *S. aureus* can be implicated in penetrating trauma and intravenous drug abuse. In immunosuppressed patients, alcoholics, and debilitated patients with diabetes, *L. monocytogenes* or *P. aeruginosa* should be considered.
- Empirical therapy for adult bacterial meningitis consists of cefotaxime or ceftriaxone. Ampicillin is added in immunosuppressed patients and in patients older than 50 years.
- Vancomycin is currently recommended in the empirical regimen to treat penicillin-resistant pneumococci.
- Rapid deterioration in patients with presumed acute bacterial meningitis has three major causes: fulminant meningitis or penicillin-resistant *S. pneumoniae* not properly covered with vancomycin, cerebral edema, and failure to diagnose empyema.

TABLE 33.1. CAUSES OF BACTERIAL
MENINGITIS

Clinical Situation	Highly Probable Organism
Otitis media, mastoiditis, sinusitis	*Streptococcus pneumoniae, Haemophilus influenzae*
Pneumonia	*S. pneumoniae, Neisseria meningitidis*
Endocarditis	*Staphylococcus aureus, S. pneumoniae*
Asplenism	*S. pneumoniae, H. influenzae, N. meningitidis*
Alcoholism	*S. pneumoniae, Listeria monocytogenes*
Cerebrospinal fluid shunt	*Staphylococcus epidermidis*
Penetrating trauma	*S. aureus*
Intravenous drug abuse	*S. aureus*
Immunosuppression, acquired immunodeficiency syndrome, and transplantation	*L. monocytogenes, Pseudomonas aeruginosa, Escherichia coli*

TABLE 33.2. INITIAL MANAGEMENT OF PATIENTS WITH ACUTE BACTERIAL MENINGITIS

Airway management	Intubation if patient has hypoxemia despite face mask with 10 L of 100% oxygen/minute, if abnormal respiratory drive or if abnormal protective reflexes (likely with motor response of withdrawal, or worse)
Mechanical ventilation	IMV/PS or CPAP mode
Blood pressure management	Maintain MAP 70–100 mm Hg
Fluid management	3 L of NaCl
	Evidence of septic shock: fluid challenges of 1L of crystalloids
	Add norepinephrine or dopamine. Vasopressin may be subsequently added to norepinephrine.
Nutrition	Enteral nutrition with continuous infusion (on day 2)
	Blood glucose control (goal 140–180 mg/dL)
Prophylaxis	DVT prophylaxis with pneumatic compression devices and SC heparin 5000 U t.i.d.

(continued)

TABLE 33.2. (CONTINUED)

	GI prophylaxis: pantoprazole 40 mg IV daily or lansoprazole 30 mg orally through nasogastric tube.
Antibiotic treatment	Cefotaxime, 2–4 g/day IV in divided doses every 12 hours, or ceftriaxone 4 g/day in divided doses every 12 hours
	Vancomycin, 20 mg/kg IV every 12 hours (trough goal 15–20 mcg/ml).
	Ampicillin, 12 g/day in divided doses every 4 hours, in immunosuppressed patients and those older than 50 years
Other measures	Dexamethasone, 10 mg IV every 6 hours for 4 days
Access	Peripheral inserted central catheter or subclavian catheter

CPAP, continuous positive airway pressure; DVT, deep vein thrombosis; GI, gastrointestinal; IMV, intermittent mandatory ventilation; IV, intravenously; MAP, mean arterial pressure; NaCl, sodium chloride; PS, pressure support; SC, subcutaneously.

TABLE 33.3. MINIMAL INHIBITORY CONCENTRATION BREAKPOINTS FOR ANTIMICROBIAL AGENTS USED TO TREAT *STREPTOCOCCUS PNEUMONIAE* INFECTIONS (MG/ML)

Antimicrobial Agent	Susceptible	Non-Susceptible Intermediate	Resistant
Penicillin	≤ 0.06	0.1–1.0	≥ 2.0
Ceftriaxone	≤ 0.5	1.0	≥ 2.0
Cefotaxime	≤ 0.5	1.0	≥ 2.0
Cefepime	≤ 0.5	1.0	≥ 2.0
Vancomycin	≤ 1.0	—	—
Rifampin	≤ 1.0	2.0	≥ 4.0
Chloramphenicol	≤ 4.0	—	≥ 8.0
Imipenem	≤ 0.12	0.25–0.5	≥ 1.0
Meropenem	≤ 0.12	≥ 0.25	—

Data from National Committee for Clinical Laboratory Standards: *Methods for Dilution Antimicrobial Susceptibility Tests for Bacteria That Grow Aerobically: Approved Standard*, 4th ed., NCCLS Document M7-A4. Wayne, PA, National Committee for Clinical Laboratory Standards, 1997.

TABLE 33.4. RECOMMENDED ANTIMICROBIAL THERAPY FOR BACTERIAL MENINGITIS

Organism	Antibiotic, Total Daily Dose (Dosing Interval)
Neisseria meningitidis	Penicillin G 24 million U/day IV in divided doses q4h *or* Aztreonam 6–8g/day IV in divided doses every 6 hours
Streptococcus pneumoniae	Cefotaxime 8–12 g/day (q4h) and vancomycin 20 mg/kg IV (q12h)
Gram-negative bacilli (except *Pseudomonas aeruginosa*)	Ceftriaxone 4 g/day IV (q12h) *or* Cefotaxime 8–12 g/day IV (q4h)
Pseudomonas aeruginosa	Ceftazidime 6–12 g/day IV (q8h)

Haemophilus influenzae type b	Ceftriaxone 4 g/day (q12h)
	or
	Cefepime 29 IV (q8h)
Staphylococcus aureus	
Methicillin-sensitive	Oxacillin 9–12 g/day IV (q4h)
Methicillin-resistant	Vancomycin 20 mg/kg IV (q12h) or nafcillin 8–12 g/day IV (q4h)
Listeria monocytogenes	Ampicillin 12 g/day IV (q4h)
Enterobacteriaceae	Cefotaxime 8–12 g/day (q4h)
	or
	Ceftriaxone 4 g/day (q12h)

TABLE 33.5. CHEMOPROPHYLAXIS
OPTIONS FOR MENINGOCOCCAL
MENINGITIS

Antibiotic	Dose
Rifampin (oral)	Adults: 600 mg q12h for 2 days
	Children > 1 month of age: 10 mg/kg q12h for 2 days
	Infant < 1 month of age: 5 mg/kg q12h for 2 days
Ciprofloxacin (oral)	Adults: 500 mg single dose; children: 125 mg
Ceftriaxone (IM)	Adults: 250 mg; children: 125 mg

IM: intramuscular.

TABLE 33.6. EMPIRICAL ANTIBIOTIC THERAPY IN SUBDURAL EMPYEMA AND EPIDURAL ABSCESS

Likely Source	Covers	Antimicrobial Therapy
Otitis media or mastoiditis	Streptococci Anaerobes Enterobacteria	Cefotaxime 8–12 g/day IV (q4h divided doses) Metronidazole 15 mg/kg loading, 7.5 mg/kg IV (q4h)
Sinusitis	Streptococci Anaerobes Enterobacteria *Staphylococcus aureus* *Haemophilus* species	*or* Piperacillin sodium and tazobactam sodium 3.375 g (q6h) IV

(a)

(b)

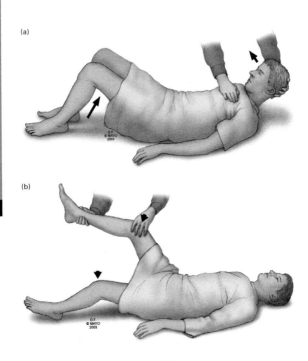

FIGURE 33.2: Brudzinski (a) and Kernig
(b) signs of meningismus.

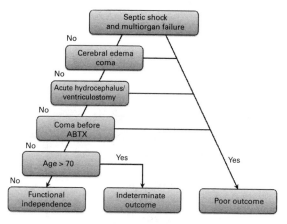

FIGURE 33.8: Outcome algorithm for bacterial meningitis. Functional independence: No assistance needed, minor handicap may remain. Indeterminate: Any statement would be a premature conclusion. Poor outcome: Severe disability or death, vegetative state.

ABTX, antibiotic therapy.

CAPSULE 33.1   PATHOGENESIS OF ACUTE BACTERIAL MENINGITIS

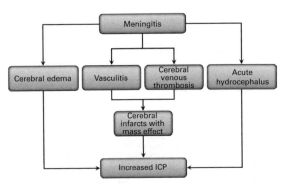

Complications of meningitis leading to increased intracranial pressure (ICP).

Chapter 34

Brain Abscess

PRACTICAL NOTES

- Medical treatment is indicated for brainstem abscess, multilocular abscesses, and surgically inaccessible deep-seated lesions.
- Surgical treatment is indicated (craniotomy or stereo-tactic aspiration) if abscesses are causing mass effect and rapid clinical deterioration. The threshold for a surgical approach should also be low if the abscess is superficially placed or in the cerebellum.
- Empirical therapy in nonimmunocompromised patients is vancomycin, cefotaxime with metronidazole.
- Empirical therapy in immunocompromised patients (particularly those infected with HIV) is indicated if multiple abscesses suggestive of toxoplasmosis are found. Therapy is guided by repeat CT scan or MRI.

TABLE 34.1. DIFFERENTIAL DIAGNOSIS
OF A SINGLE MASS SUSPICIOUS
FOR BACTERIAL ABSCESS

Noncompromised Host	Compromised Host
Cysticercosis	*Cryptococcus neoformans*
Glioma	Kaposi sarcoma
Herpes simplex	*Listeria monocytogenes*
Metastasis	Lymphoma
Multiple sclerosis	*Mycobacterium*
Sarcoidosis	*Nocardia*
	Progressive multifocal leukoencephalopathy
	Toxoplasma

TABLE 34.2. BRAIN ABSCESS: PREDISPOSING CONDITION, SITE OF ABSCESS, AND MICROBIOLOGY

Predisposing Condition	Site of Abscess	Usual Microbial Isolates
Contiguous Focus or Primary Infection		
Otitis media or mastoiditis	Temporal lobe or cerebellum	Streptococci (anaerobic or aerobic), *Bacteroides fragilis*, Enterobacteriaceae
Frontoethmoidal sinusitis	Frontal lobe	Predominantly streptococci (anaerobic or aerobic), *Bacteroides* spp., Enterobacteriaceae, *Staphylococcus aureus*, *Haemophilus* spp.
Sphenoidal sinusitis	Frontal or temporal lobe	Same as frontoethmoidal sinusitis
Periodontal abscess	Frontal lobe	Mixed *Fusobacterium*, *Bacteroides*, and *Streptococcus* spp.
Penetrating head injury or postsurgical infection	Near the laceration	*S. aureus*, streptococci, Enterobacteriaceae, *Clostridium* spp.

(continued)

TABLE 34.2. (CONTINUED)

Hematogenous Spread or Distant Site of Infection		
Congenital heart disease	Multiple sites	Streptococci (aerobic, anaerobic, or microaerophilic), *Haemophilus* spp.
Lung abscess, empyema, bronchiectasis	Multiple sites	*Fusobacterium* spp., *Actinomyces* spp., *Bacteroides* spp., *Streptococcus* spp., *Nocardia asteroides*
Bacterial endocarditis	Multiple sites	*S. aureus*, *Streptococcus* spp.

TABLE 34.3. LABORATORY STUDIES IN THE INITIAL EVALUATION OF BRAIN ABSCESS

Cultures	Blood, urine, sputum, cerebrospinal fluid
	Selected cases: gastric washings, bronchial brushing, pleural or ascitic fluid, aspirate or biopsy
Serologic studies	Viral, fungal, *Toxoplasma gondii*
Imaging studies	Chest radiograph, sinus radiograph and Panorex, electrocardiogram, echocardiography, computed tomography images of chest or abdomen

TABLE 34.4. INITIAL MANAGEMENT OF PATIENTS WITH BRAIN ABSCESS

Airway management	Intubation if patient has hypoxemia despite facemask with 10 L of 100% oxygen/minute, if abnormal respiratory drive or presence of abnormal protective reflexes (likely with motor response of withdrawal, or worse)
Mechanical ventilation	IMV/PS or CPAP mode
Fluid management	2 L of 0.9% NaCl (adjust with fever)
Nutrition	Enteral nutrition with continuous infusion (on day 2)
	Blood glucose control (goal 140–180 mg/dL)
Prophylaxis	DVT prophylaxis with pneumatic compression devices
	Consider SC heparin 5,000 U t.i.d.
	GI prophylaxis: pantoprazole 40 mg IV daily or lansoprazole 30 mg orally through nasogastric tube
	Consider seizure prophylaxis when surgery anticipated (levetiracetam 20 mg/kg IV over 60 minutes) maintenance 1,000 mg b.i.d. orally
Medical management	Third-generation cephalosporin and metronidazole
Surgical management	Aspiration with rapid deterioration, coma, mass effect, and > 3 cm
Access	Peripheral inserted central catheter

CPAP, continuous positive airway pressure; DVT, deep vein thrombosis; GI, gastrointestinal; IMV, intermittent mandatory ventilation; IV, intravenously; NaCl, sodium chloride; PS, pressure support; SC, subcutaneously.

TABLE 34.5. EMPIRICAL ANTIBIOTIC TREATMENT FOR PATIENTS WITH BRAIN ABSCESS

Nonimmunocompromised Patients

Cefotaxime	8–12 g/day IV in divided doses q4h
Metronidazole	15 mg/kg IV load; 7.5 mg/kg IV q6h
Vancomycin (with penicillin allergy)	20 mg/kg IV in divided doses q12h

Immunocompromised Patients or Those with Possible Unusual Bacterial Infection, Atypical Bacteria, or Nonbacterial Infection

Antituberculous therapy	Rifampin, 10 mg/kg/day orally
	Isoniazid, 5 mg/kg/day orally
	Pyrazinamide, 2,000 mg/day/orally
	Ethambutol, 15 mg/kg/day orally
Antifungal therapy	Amphotericin B, 0.25–1.0 mg/kg/day IV to total dose of 1.5 mg/kg/day infused over 2–6 hours

(continued)

TABLE 34.2. (CONTINUED)

Antiparasitic therapy	
Toxoplasma gondii	Pyrimethamine, initially 200 mg po and then 50–75 mg/day orally Sulfadiazine, 1–1.5 g q6h/day (leucovorin [folinic acid], 10 mg orally)
Taenia solium	Praziquantel, 60 mg/kg/day (in divided doses tid) or albendazole, 15 mg/kg/day (in divided doses tid)
Atypical bacteria	
Nocardia asteroides	Trimethoprim, sulfamethoxazole, 15 mg TMP/kg/day in 2 divided doses IV or orally qid per day or sulfisoxazole, 4–8 g/day (in 4 divided doses)

IV, intravenous.

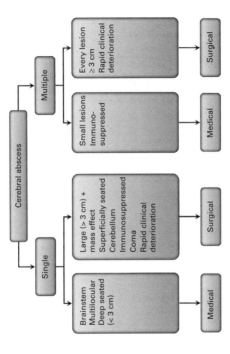

FIGURE 34.2: Guideline for management of brain abscess.

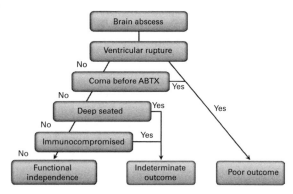

FIGURE 34.8: Outcome algorithm for brain abscess. Functional independence: No assistance needed, minor handicap may remain. Indeterminate: Any statement would be a premature conclusion. Poor outcome: Severe disability or death, vegetative state.

ABTX, antibiotic therapy.

Chapter 35

Acute Encephalitis

PRACTICAL NOTES

- Treatment of acute encephalitis is largely supportive, including seizure control and management of agitation.
- Polymerase chain reaction can reliably detect herpes simplex DNA in CSF and has largely replaced the need for brain biopsy; PCR is also available for CMV, EBV, and enteroviruses.
- Brain edema in acute viral encephalitis warrants ICP monitoring. Aggressive management, including decompressive craniectomy, may increase the chance of survival.

TABLE 35.1. ADULT EPIDEMIC VIRAL ENCEPHALITIS

Type	Virus	Severity	Mortality (%)
Eastern equine encephalomyelitis	Alphavirus	+++	50–70
Western equine encephalomyelitis	Alphavirus	++	5–10
Venezuelan equine encephalomyelitis	Alphavirus	+	< 1
Japanese encephalitis	Flavivirus	+++	25–50
St. Louis encephalitis	Flavivirus	++	70*
Murray Valley encephalitis	Flavivirus	++	10–20
Colorado tick fever	Orbivirus	+	< 1
La Crosse encephalitis	Bunyavirus	++	< 5
Lymphocytic choriomeningitis	Arenavirus	++	< 1
Argentine hemorrhagic fever	Arenavirus	++	< 10
Lassa fever	Arenavirus	++	< 15
Rabies	Rabies virus	+++	~100†
West Nile	Flavivirus	++	~70‡

* In elderly patients only
† Occasional survivors in a mildly disabled state have been reported.
‡ Experience too limited for findings to be entirely accurate
+++ Often progressing to coma
++ Variable presentation, but may be severe deficit
+ Often mild.

TABLE 35.2. INFECTIOUS DISEASES THAT CAN MASQUERADE AS VIRAL CENTRAL NERVOUS SYSTEM INFECTIONS

Bacteria
  Spirochetes
    Syphilis (secondary or meningovascular)
    Leptospirosis
  Borrelia burgdorferi infection (Lyme disease)
  Mycoplasma pneumoniae infection
  Cat-scratch fever
  Listeriosis
  Brucellosis (particularly due to *Brucella melitensis*)
  Tuberculosis
  Typhoid fever
  Parameningeal infections (epidural infection, petrositis)
  Partially treated bacterial meningitis
  Brain abscesses
  Whipple disease
Fungi
  Cryptococcosis
  Coccidioidomycosis
  Histoplasmosis
  North American blastomycosis
  Candidiasis
Parasites
  Toxoplasmosis
  Cysticercosis
  Echinococcosis
  Trichinosis
  Trypanosomiasis
  Plasmodium falciparum infection
  Amebiasis (due to *Naegleria* and *Acanthamoeba*)

Modified from Johnson RT. Acute encephalitis. *Clin Infect Dis* 1996;23:219. With permission of the University of Chicago.

TABLE 35.3. MAGNETIC RESONANCE IMAGING FINDINGS IN VIRAL ENCEPHALITIS

Site	HSE	EEE	CMV	La Crosse	St. Louis	Rabies
Frontal	X			X		
Temporal	X			X		
Basal ganglia		X				X
Thalamus		X				X
White matter			X			
Substantia nigra					X	
Meningeal enhancement			X			

CMV, cytomegalovirus; EEE, eastern equine encephalomyelitis; HSE, herpes simplex encephalitis.
X = Abnormal signal.

TABLE 35.4. MANDATORY SEROLOGIC
TESTS OF CEREBROSPINAL FLUID
IN ENCEPHALITIS OF UNKNOWN CAUSE

Herpes simplex
Cytomegalovirus
Human immunodeficiency virus
Varicella-zoster virus
Epstein-Barr virus
Toxoplasma gondii
Borrelia burgdorferi
Mycoplasma pneumoniae
Leptospira species
Legionella pneumophila
Brucella species
Syphilis
Aspergillus

TABLE 35.5. INITIAL MANAGEMENT OF ACUTE VIRAL ENCEPHALITIS

Airway management	Intubate early if deterioration is rapid. Intubation if patient has hypoxemia despite facemask with 10 L of 100% oxygen/minute, if abnormal respiratory drive or presence of abnormal protective reflexes (likely with motor response of withdrawal, or worse)
Mechanical ventilation	IMV/ PS or CPAP mode
Fluid management	Maintenance, 3 L of 0.9% NaCl (500 mL increase/°C); in patients with hyponatremia, consider dilution (treat with free-water restriction) or Addison's disease (treat with corticosteroids)
Nutrition	Enteral nutrition with continuous infusion (on day 2)
	Blood glucose control (goal 140–180 mg/dL)
Prophylaxis	DVT prophylaxis with pneumatic compression devices
	SC heparin 5,000 U t.i.d.
	GI prophylaxis: pantoprazole 40 mg IV daily or lansoprazole 30 mg orally through nasogastric tube.

Specific treatment	Antiviral: HSE: acyclovir, 10 mg/kg q8h
	CMV: ganciclovir, 5 mg/kg q12 h
	Autoimmune: PLEX/IVIG/Methylprednisolone
Other measures	Seizures: Fosphenytoin, 20 mg PE/kg followed by 300 mg IV or Levetiracetam
	20 mg/kg IV over 60 minutes. Maintenance 1,000 mg bid IV or orally
	Agitation: Midazolam (0.02 mg/kg/hr) or lorazepam (0.025 mg/kg/hr) infusion
Surgical management	Consider brain biopsy for diagnostic purposes
	Removal of necrotic temporal mass
Access	Peripheral venous catheter or Peripheral inserted central catheter

CMV, cytomegalovirus; CPAP, continuous positive airway pressure; DVT, deep vein thrombosis; GI, gastrointestinal; HSE, herpes simplex encephalitis; IMV, intermittent mandatory ventilation; IV, intravenously; IVIG, intravenous immunoglobulin; NaCl, sodium chloride; PLEX, plasma exchange; PS, pressure support; SC, subcutaneously.

TABLE 35.6. ACYCLOVIR DOSES
IN RENAL IMPAIRMENT

CRCL, mL/min*	mg/kg	Frequency
> 50	10	q8h
30–50	10	q12h
10–30	10	q24h
< 10	5	q24h

*Calculation of creatinine clearance (CRCL).

Male: $\text{CRCL}\left(\text{mL / min}\right) = \dfrac{\left(140 - \text{age}\right) \times \left(\text{ideal body weight}\left[\text{kg}\right]\right)}{\text{serum creatine}\left(\text{mg / dL}\right) \times 72}$

Female: $0.85 \times$ CRCL for men
Ideal body weight: males, 50 kg + 2.3 kg for each inch over 5 feet;
females, 45.5 kg + 2.3 kg for each inch over 5 feet.

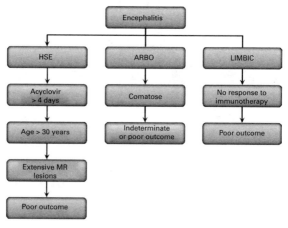

FIGURE 35.8: Outcome algorithm in viral encephalitis.
Indeterminate: Any statement would be a premature
conclusion. Functional independence: No assistance needed,
minor handicap may remain. Poor outcome: Severe disability
or death, vegetative state.

HSE, herpes simplex encephalitis.

Chapter 36

Acute Spinal Cord Disorders

PRACTICAL NOTES

- Traumatic spine injury requires not only radiologic studies but also expert evaluation.
- Magnetic resonance imaging complements clinical localization and should be performed urgently.
- Respiratory compromise and severe bradycardia should be expected in patients with complete cervical lesions.
- Methylprednisolone may be effective in traumatic SCI if administration begins within 3 hours. An intravenous bolus of 30 mg/kg is followed by infusion of 5.4 mg/kg/hr for 23 hours.
- Plasma exchange should be considered in acute demyelinating disorders not responding to corticosteroids.
- Prompt neurosurgical intervention is generally indicated for acute epidural hematoma, spinal instability from trauma or cancer destruction, and removal of a foreign object.

TABLE 36.1. BRITISH MEDICAL RESEARCH COUNCIL SCALE OF MUSCLE STRENGTH

0 No muscular contraction
1 A flicker of contraction either seen or palpated but insufficient to move a joint
2 Muscular contractions sufficient to move a joint but not against the force of gravity
3 Muscular contractions sufficient to maintain a position against the force of gravity
4 Muscular contractions sufficient to resist the force of gravity plus additional force
5 Normal motor power

Modified from *Aids to the Examination of the Peripheral Nervous System*, 4th ed. Edinburgh: W. B. Saunders, 2000. With permission of *The Guarantors of Brain*.

TABLE 36.2. AMERICAN SPINAL INJURY ASSOCIATION (ASIA) IMPAIRMENT SCALE

Grade	Description
A	Complete; no sensory or motor function preserved in the sacral segments S4–S5
B	Incomplete; sensory but not motor function preserved below the neurologic level and extending through the sacral segment S4–S5
C	Incomplete; motor function preserved below the neurologic level; most key muscles have an MRC grade 3
D	Incomplete; motor function preserved below the neurologic level; most key muscles have an MRC grade 3
E	Normal motor and sensory function

MRC, Medical Research Council.
From McDonald JW, Sadowsky C. Spinal-cord injury. *Lancet* 2002; 359:417–425. With permission of Elsevier Science.

TABLE 36.3. SPINE INSTABILITY

Cervical

- Widened interspinous space or facet joints
- Anterior listhesis > 3.5 mm
- Narrowed or widened disk space
- Focal angulation > 11 degrees
- Vertebral compression > 25%

Thoracic

- Fracture dislocation
- Posttraumatic kyphosis > 40 degrees
- Spine fractures associated with sternal fractures
- Concomitant rib fracture or costovertebral dislocation

Imhof H, Fuchsjäger M. Traumatic injuries: imaging of spinal injuries. *Eur Radiol* 2002;12:1262. With permission of Springer.

TABLE 36.4. COMMON DIAGNOSTIC CONSIDERATIONS IN ACUTE SPINAL CORD DISEASE

Disorder	Diagnostic Test
Myelopathy	
Compressive myelopathy	MRI of spine
Acute necrotic myelopathy	MRI of spine, biopsy
Vacuolar myelopathy	CSF (PMN), HIV-1
Anterior spinal artery occlusion	MRI of spine, RF, SLE, ANA
Foix-Alajouanine syndrome	MRI of spine, spinal angiogram
Radiation myelopathy	Radiation field, irradiation dose
Paraneoplastic myelopathy	CT scan of chest-abdomen, bone marrow, thyroid scan
Myelitis	
Acute disseminated encephalomyelitis	CSF (MN), MRI of brain
Postinfectious myelitis	Echovirus, coxsackievirus
Demyelinating myelitis	CSF (protein, IgG, oligoclonal bands)

Neuromyelitis optica	VEP, MRI of spine, CSF protein)
Viral myelitis	Herpes zoster, CSF (PCR), HTLV-1
Bacterial myelitis	VDRL, FTA-ABS, CSF (cells, protein)
Tropical myelitis	Circulating antigen, stools, ELISA (schistosomiasis, trichinosis)

ANA, antinuclear antibody; CSF, cerebrospinal fluid; CT, computed tomography; ELISA, enzyme-linked immunosorbent assay; FTA-ABS, fluorescent treponemal antibody absorption test; HIV, human immunodeficiency virus; MN, mononuclear leukocytes; MRI, magnetic resonance imaging; PCR, polymerase chain reaction; PMN, polymorphonuclear leukocytes; RF, rheumatoid factor; SLE, systemic lupus erythematosus; VEP, visual evoked potential.

From Berman M, Feldman S, Alter M, et al. Acute transverse myelitis: incidence and etiologic considerations. *Neurology* 1981;31:966–971; and Campi A, Filippi M, Comi G, et al. Acute transverse myelopathy: spinal and cranial MR study with clinical follow-up. *AJNR Am J Neuroradiol* 1995;16:115–123.

TABLE 36.5. INITIAL MANAGEMENT OF ACUTE SPINAL CORD DISORDER

Airway management	Incentive spirometry and assisted cough
	Intubation if patient has hypoxemia despite facemask with 10 L of 100% oxygen/minute or with abnormal respiratory drive
Mechanical ventilation	AC or IMV mode in high cervical lesions (C3–C5)
Blood pressure management	Maintain MAP 90–100 mm Hg (MAP of 85 mmHg or more for at least 7 days in traumatic spine injury) IV norepinephrine may be needed.
Fluid management	2 L of 0.9% NaCl
	Consider crystalloid infusions with shock
Nutrition	Enteral nutrition with continuous infusion (on day 2)
	Blood glucose control (goal 140–180 mg/dL)
Prophylaxis	DVT prophylaxis: Pneumatic compression devices
	SC heparin 5,000 U t.i.d.
	GI prophylaxis: Pantoprazole 40 mg daily IV or lansoprazole 30 mg orally through nasogastric tube
	Inspect skin with each turn and every 8 hours
	Bisacodyl supp and digital stimulation daily for bowel care
	Indwelling urinary catheter

Specific management	*In spinal cord compression and acute myelitis:* dexamethasone, 100 mg IV, followed by 4–25 mg/day q.i.d.
	In traumatic spine injury: Methylprednisolone < 3 hr (30 mg/kg bolus, followed by infusion of 5.4 mg/kg/hr for 23 hours); 3–8 hr (30 mg/kg bolus, followed by infusion of 5.4 mg/kg/hr for 48 hours)
Surgical management	Surgical stabilization and instrumentation in spinal cord compression from cancer
	Immediate evacuation in spinal epidural hematoma
Other measures	Consider temporary pacemaker
	Consider atropine, 0.5 mg, or isoproterenol infusion, 2–10 μg per minute
	Abdominal binders and elastic leg wraps with upright position
	Consider midodrine (2.5–10 mg orally t.i.d.) for orthostatic hypotension
	Aggressive postural drainage, rotating beds
Access	Arterial catheter to monitor blood pressures (particularly if labile blood pressures)
	Peripheral venous catheter or Peripheral inserted central catheter

AC, assist control; DVT, deep vein thrombosis; GI, gastrointestinal; IMV, intermittent mandatory ventilation; IV, intravenously; NaCl, sodium chloride; SC, subcutaneously.

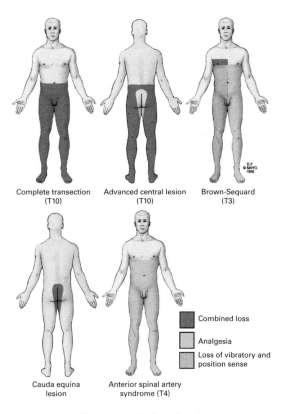

Complete transection
(T10)

Advanced central lesion
(T10)

Brown-Sequard
(T3)

Cauda equina
lesion

Anterior spinal artery
syndrome (T4)

Combined loss

Analgesia

Loss of vibratory and
position sense

FIGURE 36.1: The major spinal cord syndromes.

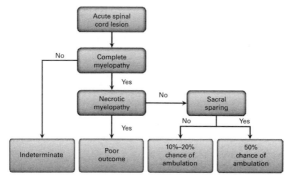

FIGURE 36.9: Algorithm of outcome in acute spinal cord disorder. Poor outcome: Severe disability or death; vegetative state. Indeterminate: Any statement would be a premature conclusion.

Chapter 37

Acute White Matter Disorders

PRACTICAL NOTES

- Progressive demyelinating disorders may need both plasma exchange and high-dose methylprednisolone to reduce morbidity.
- Acute transverse myelitis is likely not responsive to specific therapy.
- Mass effect from acute necrotic or demyelinating disease requires early ICP reduction and possible surgical evacuation.

TABLE 37.1. DISORDERS
MIMICKING ACUTE DISSEMINATED
ENCEPHALOMYELITIS

Acute viral encephalitis (arboviruses)

Herpes simplex encephalitis

Central nervous system vasculitis

Gliomatosis cerebri

Intravascular lymphoma

Progressive multifocal leukoencephalopathy

Neurosarcoidosis

Systemic lupus erythematosus

Sjögren disease

TABLE 37.2. CAUSES OF ACUTE
TRANSVERSE MYELITIS

Echovirus
Varicella
Herpes zoster
Herpes simplex virus (HSV1, HSV2)
Influenza
Epstein-Barr virus
Cytomegalovirus
Mycoplasma
Parasites (e.g., schistosomiasis)
Vaccination
Multiple sclerosis
Lupus erythematosus
Sjögren disease
Syphilis
Lyme disease

TABLE 37.3. ACUTE
LEUKOENCEPHALOPATHY IN ADULTS

Immunosuppressive agents (cyclosporine,
  tacrolimus)

Hypertensive crisis

Eclampsia, HELLP syndrome

Chemotherapeutic agents (methotrexate, 5-
fluorouracil, levamisole, intra-arterial nimustine
[ACNU])

Fulminant multiple sclerosis

Postradiation

Human immunodeficiency virus

Erythropoietin

Interferon-α

Ecstasy

Bath salts

Heroin inhalation

Progressive multifocal leukoencephalopathy

ACNU, 1-(4-amino-2-methyl-5-pyrimidinyl)-methyl-(2-chloroethyl)-
3-nitrosourea; HELLP, hemolysis, elevated liver enzymes, and low
platelet count
Data extracted from Filley CM, Kleinschmidt-deMasters BK. Toxic
encephalopathy. *N Engl J Med* 2001;345:425–432. With permission
of the publisher.

TABLE 37.4. INITIAL MANAGEMENT OF ACUTE WHITE MATTER DISORDERS

Airway management	Intubation if patient has hypoxemia despite facemask with 10 L of 100 oxygen/minute, if abnormal respiratory drive or presence of abnormal protective reflexes (likely with motor response of withdrawal, or worse)
Mechanical ventilation	IMV/PS or AC needed with high cervical cord lesions in acute transverse myelitis CPAP or PS mostly suffices for ADEM or acute leukoencephalopathies
Fluid management	2 L of 0.9% NaCl per 24 hours
Nutrition	Enteral nutrition with continuous infusion (on day 2) Blood glucose control (goal 140–180 mg/dL)
Prophylaxis	DVT prophylaxis with pneumatic compression devices SC heparin 5,000 U t.i.d. GI prophylaxis: Pantoprazole 40 mg IV daily or lansoprazole 30 mg orally through nasogastric tube

(continued)

TABLE 37.4. (CONTINUED)

Other measures	IV methylprednisone 1 g/day for 3–5 days
	Series of plasma exchanges (7–10) or series of IV immunoglobulin 0.4 g/kg/day for 5 days
	Discontinue chemotherapy (if applicable)
	Substitute immunosuppression with sirolimus (if applicable)
Access	Peripheral venous catheter or peripheral inserted central catheter

AC, assist control; ADEM, acute disseminated encephalomyelitis; CPAP, continuous positive airway pressure; DVT, deep vein thrombosis; GI, gastrointestinal; IMV, intermittent mandatory ventilation; IV, intravenously; NaCl, sodium chloride; PS, pressure support; SC, subcutaneously.

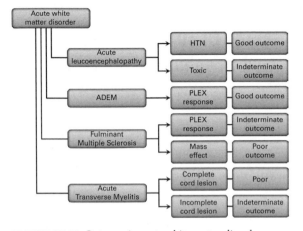

FIGURE 37.11 Outcome in acute white matter disorders.

ADEM, acute disseminated encephalomyelitis; HTN, hypertension;
PLEX, plasma exchange.

Chapter 38

Acute Obstructive Hydrocephalus

PRACTICAL NOTES

- Acute obstructive hydrocephalus may be life-threatening and in many circumstances requires an urgent ventriculostomy.
- Primary intraventricular hemorrhage and acute hydrocephalus may need additional treatment with thrombolytics.
- Treatment of acute hydrocephalus often comes first, followed by management of the obstructing tumor.
- Ventriculostomy may need to be internalized. Some patients require no valve or a low-pressure valve to maintain a normal ventricular size.

TABLE 38.1. MASSES CAUSING ACUTE OBSTRUCTIVE HYDROCEPHALUS

Type	CT Scan Characteristics	Treatment
Intraventricular tumors		
Colloid cyst	Rounded, anterior 3V, widened SP, collapse of posterior 3V, ID, or HYP	Surgery or stereotactic aspiration
Plexus papilloma	Oval, 4V, LV, HYP	Total excision
Ependymoma	Lobulated, 4V, LV, ID	Excision and radiotherapy
Oligodendroglioma	Lobulated, LV, HYP, calcification	Resection
Ganglioglioma	3V, ID, HYP	Resection
Astrocytoma	LV, HD or HYP, irregular shape	Radiation, resection
Epidermoid cyst	4V, HYP, ID	Resection
Masses in pineal region		
Pineoblastoma	Lobulated, HD at peripheral rim, calcifications	Resection, radiation
Germinoma	ID, rounded	Radiation
Teratoma	HD or HYP, calcifications, lipid content	Resection
Vein of Galen aneurysm	HYP, rounded, triangular	Endovascular occlusion

CT, computed tomography; HD, hypodense; HYP, hyperdense; ID, isodense; LV, lateral ventricle; SP, septum pellucidum; 3V, third ventricle; 4V, fourth ventricle.
Data obtained from references 2, 17, 21, 22, 33, 35.

TABLE 38.2. INITIAL MANAGEMENT OF ACUTE HYDROCEPHALUS

Airway management	Protect airway with nasal trumpet or intubate if patient has hypoxemia despite facemask with 10 L of 100 oxygen/minute or if abnormal respiratory drive or if abnormal protective reflexes (likely with motor response of withdrawal, or worse)
Mechanical ventilation	CPAP mode
	IMV/PS may be needed in obstructing lesions in the posterior fossa
Fluid management	2 L of 0.9% NaCl
Nutrition	Enteral nutrition with continuous infusion (on day 2)
	Blood glucose control (goal 140–180 mg/dL)
Prophylaxis	DVT prophylaxis with pneumatic compression devices
	SC heparin 5,000 U t.i.d.
	GI prophylaxis: Pantoprazole 40 mg IV daily or lansoprazole 30 mg orally through nasogastric tube
Surgical management	Ventriculostomy at 5–10 cm H_2O
	Revision prior shunt
	Ventricular peritoneal shunt (pressure valve varies)
	Surgical extirpation of obstructing mass
Access	Peripheral venous catheter or peripheral inserted central catheter

CPAP, continuous positive airway pressure; DVT, deep vein thrombosis; GI, gastrointestinal; IMV, intermittent mandatory ventilation; IV, intravenously; NaCl, sodium chloride; PS, pressure support; SC, subcutaneously.

CAPSULE 38.1 PATHOPHYSIOLOGY OF ACUTE HYDROCEPHALUS

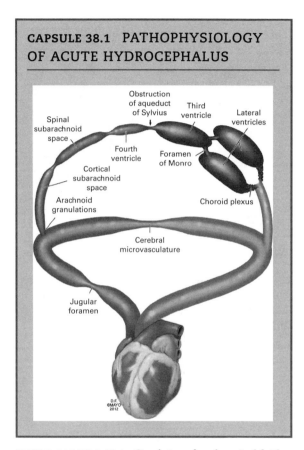

FIGURE CAPSULE 38.1: Circulation of cerebrospinal fluid.

(adapted from Sakka L, Coll G, Chazal J. Anatomy and physiology of cerebrospinal fluid. *Eur Ann Otorhinolaryngol Head Neck Dis* 2011; 128:309–316.

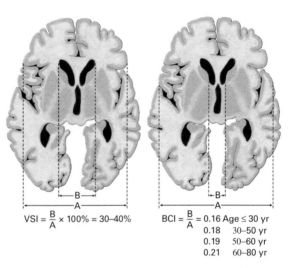

FIGURE 38.6: Measurement on computed tomographic scan of the ventricular system in acute hydrocephalus. Numbers indicate normal values. The ventricular size index (VSI) is not corrected for age.

BCI, bicaudate index.

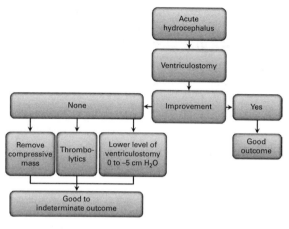

FIGURE 38.7: Outcome prediction in acute obstructive hydrocephalus. Good outcome: No assistance needed, minor handicap may remain. Indeterminate outcome: Any statement would be a premature conclusion.

Chapter 39

Malignant Brain Tumors

PRACTICAL NOTES

- Patients in NICU with a recent malignant brain tumor need close monitoring for seizures, post-debulking cerebral edema or hemorrhage and control of airway.
- Dexamethasone may rapidly reduce clinical signs of mass effect.
- Status epilepticus (epilepsia partialis continua) does occur with recurrence and may need surgical resection or anesthetic drugs

TABLE 39.1. INITIAL MANAGEMENT OF MALIGNANT BRAIN TUMOR

Airway management	Intubation when patient's consciousness declines, and if abnormal protective reflexes (likely with motor response of withdrawal, or worse)
	Tracheostomy for brainstem tumors
Mechanical ventilation	Usually CPAP or IMV/PS
Fluids management	2L of 0.9% NaCl
Nutrition	Enteral nutrition with continuous infusion (on day 2)
	Blood glucose control (goal 140–180 mg/dL)
Prophylaxis	DVT prophylaxis with pneumatic compression devices
	Consider SC heparin 5000 U t.i.d.
	GI prophylaxis: Pantoprazole 40 mg IV daily or lansoprazole 30 mg orally through nasogastric tube
	Administration of trimethoprim-sulfamethoxazole DS (160 mg) in patients with dexamethasone

(continued)

TABLE 39.1. CONTINUED

Specific management	Levetiracetam 1,000 mg IV over 15 minutes and 1,000 mg bid maintenance
	Bolus administration of dexamethasone (10 mg intravenously)
	Maintenance dexamethasone (8–16 mg/day)
Access	Peripheral venous catheter or peripheral inserted central catheter
Surgical treatment	Debulking procedure
	Stereotactic biopsy

CPAP, continuous positive airway pressure; DVT, deep vein thrombosis; GI, gastrointestinal; IMV, intermittent mandatory ventilation; IV, intravenous; LMWH, low-molecular-weight heparin; NaCl, sodium chloride; PS, pressure support; SC, subcutaneous.

TABLE 39.2. CURRENT TREATMENT OF MALIGNANT GLIOMAS

Type of Tumor	Treatment
Newly diagnosed tumors	
Glioblastomas (WHO grade IV)	Maximal surgical resection, plus radiotherapy plus concomitant and adjuvant TMZ or carmustine wafers
Angioplastic astrocytomas (WHO grade III)	Maximal surgical resection, TMZ alone, or radiotherapy plus concomitant and adjuvant TMZ
Anaplastic oligodendrogliomas and anaplastic oligoastrocytoma (WHO grade III)	Maximal surgical resection, radiotherapy alone, TMZ or PVC with or without radiotherapy afterward, radiotherapy plus concomitant and adjuvant TMZ, or radiotherapy plus adjuvant TMZ
Recurrent tumors	Reoperation in selected patients, carmustine wafers, conventional chemotherapy (e.g., lomustine PCV, carmustine PCV, carboplatin, irinotecan hydrochloride, etoposide phosphate, bevacizumab plus irinotecan), experimental therapies

PCV, procarbazine; TMZ, temozolomide; WHO, World Health Organization.
Adapted from Wen PY, Kesari S. Malignant gliomas in adults. *N Engl J Med* 2008;359:492–507. Used with permission.

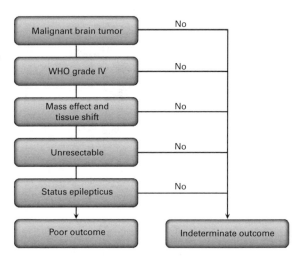

FIGURE 39.5: Outcome in malignant brain tumors. Poor outcome: Severe disability or death, negative state. Indeterminate outcome: Any statement would be a premature conclusion.

Chapter 40

Status Epilepticus

PRACTICAL NOTES

- One can expect that a large proportion of patients with status epilepticus can be controlled with benzodiazepines (lorazepam 4–8 mg) and an adequate loading dose of (fos)phenytoin (20 mg/kg).
- Recurrence of seizures after adequate phenytoin loading could be treated with midazolam or propofol infusion.
- If all else fails, intravenous administration of ketamine, pentobarbital, isoflurane, or electroconvulsive therapy should be considered.
- Outcome of status epilepticus is strongly related to the response to the first dose of antiepileptic agent and to the underlying trigger.

TABLE 40.1. PHARMACEUTICAL AGENTS USED IN THE NICU THAT CAN REDUCE SEIZURE THRESHOLD

Antibiotics	Imipenem
	Norfloxacin
	Ciprofloxacin
	Cefepime
	Penicillin derivatives
Antidepressants	Amitriptyline
	Doxepin
	Nortriptyline
	Fluoxetine, sertraline
Antipsychotics	Chlorpromazine
	Haloperidol
	Thioridazine
	Perphenazine
	Trifluoperazine

TABLE 40.2. INITIAL MANAGEMENT OF STATUS EPILEPTICUS

Airway management	Intubation if patient has hypoxemia despite facemask with 10 L of 100% oxygen/minute, if abnormal respiratory drive or if abnormal protective reflexes (likely with motor response of withdrawal, or worse)
	Elective endotracheal intubation if second-line treatment (propofol or midazolam) is anticipated
Mechanical ventilation	IMV/PS
	AC with use of anesthetic drugs
Fluid management	2–3 L of 0.9% NaCl; increase with fever or evidence of rhabdomyolysis
Nutrition	Enteral nutrition with continuous infusion (on day 2)
	Blood glucose control (goal 140–180 mg/dL)
Prophylaxis	DVT prophylaxis with pneumatic compression devices
	SC heparin 5,000 U t.i.d.
	GI prophylaxis: pantoprazole 40 mg IV daily or lansoprazole 30 mg orally through nasogastric tube.
	Consider β-blockade or diltiazem infusion in patients with persistent rapid ventricular rate

(continued)

TABLE 40.2. CONTINUED

Specific management	Lorazepam, 4 mg (total dose, 8 mg)
	Phenytoin loading, 20 mg/kg (rate, 50 mg/min or, in elderly, 25 mg/min), or fosphenytoin, 20 mg PE/kg (rate 100–150 mg PE/min)
	If unsuccessful (recurrent clinical seizure or electrographic seizures) proceed with IV midazolam bolus 0.2 mg/kg, start 0.1 mg/kg/hr and increase until seizures stop
Access	Two large-bore intravenous catheters
	Peripheral inserted central catheter or internal jugular central venous line if vasopressors are needed or anticipated

AC, assist control; DVT, deep vein thrombosis; GI, gastrointestinal; IMV, intermittent mandatory ventilation; IV, intravenously; NaCl, sodium chloride; PE, phenytoin equivalents; PS, pressure support; SC, subcutaneously.

TABLE 40.3. INTRAVENOUS ANTIEPILEPTIC AGENTS USED TO TREAT CONVULSIVE STATUS EPILEPTICUS

Drug	Initial Dose (Bolus)	Rate	Infusion (Maintenance)	Precautions
Midazolam	0.2 mg/kg	< 4 mg/min	0.1–0.6 mg/kg/hr	Mechanical ventilation invariably needed; vasopressors for hypotension
Lorazepam	4 mg	1–2 mg/min		Cardiac monitoring for cardiac arrhythmias (bradycardia)
Phenytoin	18–20 mg/kg	50 mg/min		Cardiac and blood pressure monitoring
Fosphenytoin	18–20 mg PE/kg	100–150 mg PE/min		Cardiac and blood pressure monitoring

(*continued*)

TABLE 40.3. CONTINUED

Drug	Initial Dose (Bolus)	Rate	Infusion (Maintenance)	Precautions
Phenobarbital	10–20 mg/kg	30–50 mg/min	1–3 mg/kg/hr	Mechanical ventilation with high dose (> 40 mg/kg) may be needed
Pentobarbital	10–15 mg/kg	1–2 hours	1–3 mg/kg/hr	Vasopressors for hypotension
Lidocaine	1.5–2 mg/kg	< 50 mg/min	3 mg/kg/hr	Cardiac monitoring (bradycardia, heart block)
Isoflurane	Inhalation to MAC (0.8%–1.1%)			Full anesthetic system and anesthesia support

Propofol	2 mg/kg initially	Slow push	1–5 mg/kg/hr	Vasopressors for hypotension (monitoring for metabolic acidosis)
Ketamine	1 mg/kg	2 min	10–50 mg/kg/min	Tachyphylaxis (increasing dose needed)
Valproate	20–30 mg/kg	20 mg/min	1–4 mg/kg/hr	Monitoring of albumin

MAC, minimum alveolar concentration; PE, phenytoin equivalents.

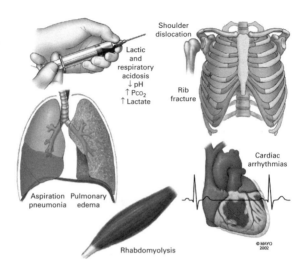

FIGURE 40.1: Systemic effects of status epilepticus.

From Wijdicks EFM. The multifaceted care of status epilepticus. *Epilepsia* 2013;54 Suppl 6:61–63.

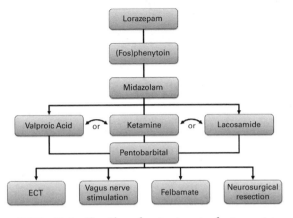

FIGURE 40.4: Algorithm for treatment-refractory status epilepticus.

ECT, electro-convulsive therapy.

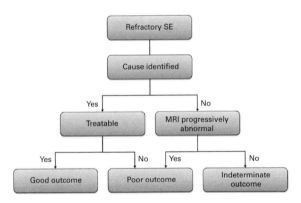

FIGURE 40.5: Outcome algorithm for status epilepticus. Poor outcome: Severe disability or death, vegetative state. Functional independence: No assistance needed, minor handicap may remain.

Chapter 41

Traumatic Brain Injury

PRACTICAL NOTES

- Intracranial pressure monitoring is strongly indicated in comatose patients with TBI, are usually patients with brain swelling or multiple contusions on CT scan, and in patients who need sedation or neuromuscular blockade to control mechanical ventilation.
- Mannitol or hypertonic saline are used to reduce ICP. Brief hyperventilation may be useful if ICP is not controlled. Alternatively, propofol, barbiturate treatment, or decompressive craniotomy are measures of last resort with unproven efficacy.
- Bilateral fixed, dilated pupils in patients with traumatic hematomas alone are a sign of poor prognosis, but 25% of patients may recover with independent function. Outcome is much worse in patients who additionally have bilateral extensor posturing.
- Poor outcome is expected in comatose elderly patients, and in those with abnormal pupils, hypoxemia or shock on admission, or multiple contusions on CT scans.
- Outcome is very difficult to predict accurately in younger individuals.

TABLE 41.1. TYPES OF COMPUTED TOMOGRAPHY SCAN ABNORMALITIES IN TRAUMATIC BRAIN INJURY

Intraparenchymal
    Diffuse axonal injury
    Diffuse brain swelling
    Hemorrhagic contusion
    Tissue tear (shear) hemorrhage
    Brainstem hemorrhage
Extra-axial compartment
    Subarachnoid hemorrhage (sulci, vertex)
    Intraventricular
    Subdural hematoma
    Epidural hematoma
Secondary lesions
    Watershed, cortex, globi pallidi and thalami
        infarcts (anoxic–ischemic injury)
    Posterior cerebral artery territory infarct
        (brainstem displacement)
    Middle cerebral artery territory infarct (traumatic
        carotid dissection)

TABLE 41.2. INITIAL MANAGEMENT OF TRAUMATIC BRAIN INJURY

Airway management	Intubation if patient has hypoxemia despite facemask with 10 L of 100% oxygen/minute, if abnormal respiratory drive or if abnormal protective reflexes (likely with motor response of withdrawal, or worse)
	Emergency tracheostomy in major facial injury
Mechanical ventilation	IMV/PS
	AC if pulmonary contusion or aspiration. Increasing PEEP if gas exchange is inadequate
	Chest tube in traumatic pneumothorax
Fluid management	0.9% NaCl, 3 L/day
Blood pressure management	Labetalol, 10–20 mg IV, for persistent hypertension (mean arterial pressure > 130 mm Hg); hydralazine 10–20 mg IV if bradycardia
Nutrition	Enteral nutrition with continuous infusion (on day 2)
	Blood glucose control (goal 140–180 mg/dL).

Prophylaxis	DVT prophylaxis with pneumatic compression devices and SC heparin 5,000 U t.i.d. Consider preventive IVC filter placement
	GI prophylaxis: pantoprazole 40 mg IV daily or lansoprazole 30 mg orally through nasogastric tube
ICP management	Placement of ICP monitoring device when comatose, ICH or brain swelling on CT or need for neuromuscular blockade.
	CPP > 70 mm Hg; ICP < 20 mm Hg
	Head elevation, 30°
	Mannitol, 0.25–1 g/kg, or hypertonic saline 23% 30 mL.
	Consider brief periods of hyperventilation
	Normothermia or induced hypothermia
Surgical management	Consider decompressive hemicraniectomy or bilateral frontal craniectomies with refractory ICP
	Consider evacuation of contusional mass

(continued)

TABLE 41.2. CONTINUED

Additional measures	No corticosteroids (unless additional spinal cord lesion)
	Consider levetiracetam 1,000 mg IV over 15 minutes, 1,000 mg b.i.d. maintenance for 7 days
	Consider nimodipine, 60 mg q6h, for traumatic SAH
	Arterial catheter to monitor blood pressure (if IV antihypertensive drugs anticipated)
Access	Peripheral venous catheter or peripheral inserted central catheter

CPP, cerebral perfusion pressure; CT, computed tomography; DVT, deep vein thrombosis; GCS, Glasgow coma scale; GI, gastrointestinal; ICH, intracranial hemorrhage; ICP, intracranial pressure; IMV, intermittent mandatory ventilation; MAP, mean arterial pressure; NaCl, sodium chloride; PEEP, positive end-expiratory pressure; PS, pressure support; SAH, subarachnoid hemorrhage.

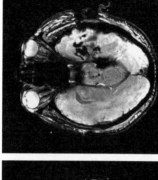

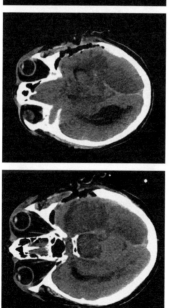

FIGURE 41.13: MRI showing secondary infarction in the PCA territory (thalamus and parietooccipital region) as a result of brain tissue shift (in this example, acute epidural hematoma).

Chapter 42

Guillain-Barré Syndrome

PRACTICAL NOTES

- Absolute indications for intensive care admission are recent 30% reduction in pulmonary function variables (vital capacity, PI_{max}, PE_{max}), oropharyngeal weakness, evidence of aspiration on chest radiographs, and dysautonomia.
- Intubation and mechanical ventilation are indicated in patients with vital capacity less than 20 mL, PI_{max} less than –30 cm H_2O, and PE_{max} less than 40 cm H_2O ("20–30–40 rule"); hypoxemia; and rapid shallow breathing.
- IVIG (0.4 g/kg/day for 5 days) or plasma exchange (albumin 5% as replacement fluid) of 250 mL/kg in five sessions on alternate days can be instituted, and they are equally effective.
- Tracheostomy may be delayed at least 2 weeks awaiting improvement from specific therapy. If there is evidence of the axonal form of GBS or significant bulbar weakness causing marked discomfort in handling secretions, tracheostomy can be placed earlier.
- Blood pressure changes could be a result of dysautonomia. Drugs used to treat blood pressure may cause exaggerated effects. Complete heart block is rare, and a temporary pacemaker may be necessary. Patients should be closely monitored for development of adynamic ileus.

TABLE 42.1. CLINICAL FEATURES OF GBS, MFS AND THEIR SUBTYPES

Category	Clinical features		
	Pattern of weakness	Ataxia	Hypersomnolence
GBS			
Classic GBS	Four limbs	No or minimal	No
Pharyngeal–cervical–brachial weakness*	Bulbar, cervical and upper limbs	No	No
Acute pharyngeal weakness‡	Bulbar	No	No
Paraparetic GBS*	Lower limbs	No	No
Bifacial weakness with paraesthesias*	Facial	No	No
MFS			
Classic MFS	Ophthalmoplegia	Yes	No
Acute ophthalmoparesis§	Ophthalmoplegia	No	No
Acute ataxic neuropathy§	No weakness	Yes	No

(continued)

TABLE 42.1. CONTINUED

Category	Clinical features		
	Pattern of weakness	Ataxia	Hypersomnolence
Acute ptosis§	Ptosis	No	No
Acute mydriasis§	Paralytic mydriasis	No	No
BBE‖	Ophthalmoplegia	Yes	Yes
Acute ataxic hypersomnolence	No weakness	Yes	Yes

*Localized subtypes of GBS. ‡Incomplete form of pharyngeal–cervical–brachial weakness. §Incomplete forms of MFS. ¶Incomplete form of BBE. Abbreviations: BBE, Bickerstaff brainstem encephalitis; GBS, Guillain–Barré syndrome; MFS, Miller Fisher syndrome.
Adapted from Wakerly et al. [116,117]

TABLE 42.2. ANTIBODIES ASSOCIATED
WITH CLINICAL VARIANTS
OF GUILLAIN-BARRÉ SYNDROME

Clinical Manifestation	Ganglioside and Galactocerebroside Antibodies
Acute motor and axonal neuropathy (AMSAN)	GM, GM_{1b}, GD_{1a}
Acute motor axonal neuropathy (AMAN)	GM, GM_{1b}, GD_{1a}, Gal Nac-GD_{1a}
Acute sensory neuropathy	GD_{1b}
Ropper's regional variants	GT_{1a}
Fisher's variant	GD_{1b}, GT_{1a}

Adapted from Hughes RAC, Cornblath DR. Guillain-Barré syndrome. *Lancet* 2005; 366:1653–1666. With permission of publisher.

TABLE 42.3. DISORDERS FREQUENTLY MIMICKING GUILLAIN-BARRÉ SYNDROME

Disease	Relevant Clinical Features	Helpful Laboratory Tests
Transverse myelitis	Sensory level Urinary incontinence No facial or bulbar involvement	MRI of spine with gadolinium CSF: pleocytosis (> 200 cells)
Myasthenia gravis	Marked fatiguing ptosis and ophthalmoplegia Intact tendon reflexes Masseter weakness No dysautonomia	EMG, NCV, repetitive stimulation Normal CSF Neostigmine test
Vasculitic neuropathy	History of PAN, SLE, WG, RA Pain without paresthesias Marked asymmetry of weakness	Chest and sinus radiographs or CT scan of thorax Nerve and muscle biopsies
Carcinomatous or lymphomatous meningitis	Cognitive changes or stupor Radicular pain Asymmetrical cranial nerve involvement	CSF cytology MRI with gadolinium MRI of spine or brain with gadolinium

CSF, cerebrospinal fluid; CT, computed tomography; EMG, electromyography; MRI, magnetic resonance imaging; NCV, nerve conduction velocity; PAN, polyarteritis nodosa; RA, rheumatoid arthritis; SLE, systemic lupus erythematosus; WG, Wegener's granulomatosis.

TABLE 42.4. ELECTRODIAGNOSTIC
FINDINGS IN 113 CONSECUTIVE
PATIENTS WITH GUILLAIN-BARRÉ
SYNDROME*

Patient Findings	No.	%
PCB and DL	30	27
Isolated PCB	31	27
Generalized slowing	25	22
PCB and DCB	11	10
Isolated DL	6	5
PCB and ICB	4	4
Absent response	2	2
PCB, ICB, and DL	1	1
DL and ICB	1	1
Isolated ICB	1	1
Normal†	1	1
Total‡	113	

*The major motor nerve abnormalities were categorized as follows:
Distal lesion (DL): > 15% increase in duration of compound muscle
action potential (CMAP) or increased distal motor latency on distal stimulation, with motor nerve conduction velocity > 80% of the
lower limit of normal.
Distal conduction block (DCB): decreased CMAP amplitude
(median or ulnar CMAP, < 4,000 mV; peroneal or tibial CMAP, <
2,000mV) in at least two nerves, with normal motor nerve conduction velocity, duration of CMAP, and distal motor latency.
Proximal conduction block (PCB): absent F waves or decreased F-
wave persistence in the presence of motor nerve conduction velocity > 80% of the lower limit of normal, and no distal or intermediate
block in the same nerve.
Intermediate conduction block (ICB): > 40% reduction between distal (D) and proximal (P) stimulation sites, specifically in the following ratio: [CMAP (D) − CMAP (P)]/[CMAP (D)] × 100, with <
10% difference in duration between sites without distal conduction
block, increased duration, or distal motor latency in the same nerve.
Generalized slowing: maximum motor conduction velocity < 80%
of the lower limit of normal in at least two of the median, ulnar,
peroneal, or tibial nerves.
Absent response: no evoked motor response with distal stimulation
sites in at least three nerves.

(*continued*)

Multiple abnormalities: a combination of two or more of abnormalities 1 through 4, above.

Denervation: at least two muscles in the arms and two in the legs were examined for spontaneous activity in the form of fibrillation potentials or positive sharp deflections.

† Prolonged F-wave latencies were found on repeated testing 2 days later.

‡ Electromyography demonstrated extensive fibrillation in 10 patients.

Source: Ropper AH, Wijdicks EFM, Shahani BT. Electrodiagnostic abnormalities in 113 consecutive patients with Guillain-Barré syndrome. *Arch Neurol* 1990;47:881–887. With permission of the American Medical Association.

TABLE 42.5. INITIAL MANAGEMENT OF GUILLAIN-BARRÉ SYNDROME

Airway management	Intubation with hypoxemia and rapid shallow breathing
	Intubation if vital capacity < 20 mL/kg and maximum inspiratory pressure ≤ −30 cm H_2O and maximum expiratory pressure < 40 cm H_2O
	Tracheostomy in most patients, but may defer if improvement is seen with PLEX or IVIG
Mechanical ventilation	IMV/PS or AC if severe atelectasis
Fluid management	2 L of 0.9% NaCl
Nutrition	Full strength enteral nutrition
	Early PEG in mechanically ventilated patients
	TPN with adynamic ileus
Sleep enhancement	Melatonin, zolpidem, doxylamine
Prophylaxis	DVT prophylaxis with pneumatic compression devices
	SC heparin 5,000 U t.i.d.
	GI prophylaxis: pantoprazole 40 mg daily IV or lansoprazole 30 mg orally through nasogastric tube

(continued)

TABLE 42.5. CONTINUED

Specific management	IVIG, 0.4 g/kg/day for 5 days
	PLEX on 5 alternate days for a total of 250 mL/kg, if IVIG is not tolerated
Other measures	Oxycodone, fentanyl, or tramadol for pain
	Aggressive skin care
	Physical therapy and splinting to prevent contractures
Access	Arterial catheter to monitor blood pressures (if IV antihypertensive drugs anticipated)
	Peripheral venous catheter and place high flow catheter with PLEX

AC, assist control; DVT, deep vein thrombosis; GI, gastrointestinal; IMV, intermittent mandatory ventilation; IV, intravenously; IVIG, intravenous immunoglobulin; NaCl, sodium chloride; PLEX, plasma exchange; PS, pressure support; TPN, total parenteral nutrition; SC, subcutaneously.

TABLE 42.6. COMPLICATIONS DURING AND AFTER PLASMA EXCHANGE

Complication	Potential Causes	Management
Hypocalcemia	Citrate	Prophylactic calcium administration ($CaCl_2$) 1 gram in 50 mL of normal saline, rate 30 minutes in central line
Hemorrhage	Depletion of coagulation factors by albumin	2 units of fresh frozen plasma (400–500 mL) at end of each exchange
Anaphylaxis or sensitivity	Anti-IgA antibodies Prekallikrein activator or bradykinin ACE-I*	Diagnostic evaluation after premedication with prednisone, 50 mg orally 13, 7, and 1 hour before treatment; diphenhydramine, 50 mg orally 1 hour before treatment; ephedrine, 25 mg orally 1 hour before treatment and before pheresis

(continued)

TABLE 42.6. CONTINUED

Complication	Potential Causes	Management
Thrombocytopenia	Filter thrombosis Centrifugal methods	Plasma separation is substituted
Hypovolemia or hypotension	Inadequate or hypooncotic volume replacement Cardiac arrhythmia Dysautonomia	5% albumin, continuous flow separations with matched input and output
Hypothermia	Cold replacement fluids	Warming of fluids
Hypokalemia	Albumin devoid of potassium	Add 4 mEq of potassium to each liter of 5% albumin

IgA, immunoglobulin A.
* Angiotensin I—converting enzyme inhibitors (ACE-I) should be held 72 hours before plasma exchange

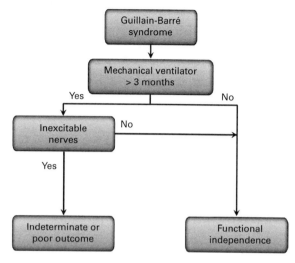

FIGURE 42.5: Outcome algorithm in Guillain-Barré syndrome. Indeterminate: Any statement would be a premature conclusion. Poor outcome: Severe disability and chance of fatal outcome from complications. Functional independence: No assistance needed, minor handicap may remain.

Chapter 43

Myasthenia Gravis

PRACTICAL NOTES

- Myasthenic crisis is mostly triggered by intercurrent infection, recent tapering off or first-time initiation of corticosteroids, and elective surgery. Initial steps in management of severe cases are endotracheal intubation, mechanical ventilation, discontinuation of pyridostigmine therapy, and plasma exchange. Bilevel positive airway pressure ventilation may prevent endotracheal intubation in some patients.
- Cholinergic symptoms are characterized by miosis, thick bronchial secretions, muscle fasciculations, abdominal cramping, diarrhea, and tearing. Bronchospasm, aspiration, or difficulty in clearing very thick secretions may cause respiratory failure.
- If a myasthenic crisis has not abated after 5 days of plasma exchange, prednisone (1 mg/kg/day) should be started or increased. Cyclosporine (5 mg/kg) or mycophenolate mofetil (1 gram bid) should be considered when treatment fails.
- Postoperative deterioration in myasthenia gravis can be largely eliminated by preoperative plasma exchange and postoperative pain control with fentanyl.

TABLE 43.1. CLINICAL EXAMINATION OF MYASTHENIA GRAVIS

Examine for ptosis (60 sec)
Diplopia lateral gaze (60 sec)
Eyelid closure or total ptosis
Dysarthria counting 1–50
Biting on tongue depressor, pushing away with tongue
Swallowing ½ cup water
Arm outstretched at 90° supine (90 sec)
Head lift 45° supine (120 sec)
Legs outstretched at 45° supine (100 sec)
Counting one breath to 20
Accessory muscles used

* Partly based on quantitative myasthenia gravis score

TABLE 43.2. DIAGNOSTIC TESTS IN MYASTHENIA GRAVIS

Electromyography, nerve conduction velocity, repetitive stimulation, single fiber study
Edrophonium or neostigmine test
Acetylcholine receptor blocking antibodies, titin antibodies, muscle antibodies
Thyroid, parietal cell antibodies
Thyroxine, triiodothyronine, thyrotropin
Computed tomography scan of the chest
Serial arterial blood gas determinations
Serial measurements of vital capacity and maximal inspiratory pressure
Preoperative pulmonary function test (with neostigmine provocation, optional)

TABLE 43.3. INITIAL MANAGEMENT OF PATIENTS WITH MYASTHENIC CRISIS

Airway management	Endotracheal intubation in patients with impaired swallowing mechanism leading to inability to clear secretions, ineffective cough and nasal voice, signs of aspiration pneumonitis on chest radiograph, any patient with marginal Pao_2, widening A–a gradient, or any vital capacity near 15 mL/kg Tracheostomy deferred
Mechanical ventilation	BiPAP trial (if no hypercapnia) IMV/PS
Nutrition	Enteral nutrition with continuous infusion (day 2)
Prophylaxis	DVT prophylaxis with pneumatic compression devices SC heparin 5,000 U t.i.d. GI prophylaxis: Pantoprazole 40 mg IV daily or lansoprazole 30 mg orally through nasogastric tube
Specific management	Plasma exchange: 5 plasma exchanges or 5 days of IVIG, 0.4 g/kg/day; 2 consecutive days of plasma exchange are followed by three exchanges on alternate days

	Prednisone (60 mg/day) is given if no improvement after 5 days of plasma exchange
Other measures	Pyridostigmine is stopped during mechanical ventilation
	Pyridostigmine therapy is gradually reinstated intravenously or intramuscularly
Access	Peripheral venous catheter and place high-flow catheter with plasma exchange

A–a, alveolar–arterial; BiPAP, bilevel positive airway pressure ventilation; DVT, deep vein thrombosis; GI, gastrointestinal; IMV, intermittent mandatory ventilation; IV, intravenously; IVIG, intravenous immunoglobulin; PS, pressure support; SC, subcutaneously.

TABLE 43.4. PHARMACEUTICAL AGENTS WITH THE POTENTIAL TO AGGRAVATE MYASTHENIA GRAVIS

Antibiotics	*Cardiovascular Agents*	*Miscellaneous*
Clindamycin	Quinidine	Penicillamine
Colistin	Propranolol	Chloroquine
Kanamycin	Procainamide	Succinylcholine
Neomycin	Practolol	Curare and other relaxants
Streptomycin	Lidocaine	Decamethonium
Tobramycin	Verapamil	Phenytoin
Tetracyclines	Nifedipine	Trimethadione
Gentamicin	Diltiazem	Carbamazepine
Polymyxin B		
Bacitracin	*Psychotropic agents*	
Trimethoprim-sulfamethoxazole	Chlorpromazine	
	Promazine	

Hormones

ACTH	Phenelzine
Corticosteroids	Lithium
Thyroid hormone	Diazepam
Oral contraceptives	

ACTH, adrenocorticotrophic hormone.

TABLE 43.5. CHOLINESTERASE
INHIBITOR DOSES
IN MYASTHENIA GRAVIS

	Oral (mg)	Intravenous (mg)
Pyridostigmine bromide (Mestinon)	60	2.0
Neostigmine bromide (Prostigmin)	15	NA
Neostigmine methylsulfate (Prostigmin)	NA	0.5

NA, not available.

TABLE 43.6. DIFFERENTIATION OF CHOLINERGIC AND MYASTHENIC CRISES

	Cholinergic Crises	Myasthenic Crises
Frequency*	Rare	Common
Trigger	Overdose, drug therapy for MG	Infection, certain drugs, corticosteroids
Pupils	Miosis	Mydriasis
Respiration	Bronchus plugging and spasm, marked salivation	Diaphragm weakness
Fasciculations, cramps	Present	Absent
Diarrhea	Present	Absent

MG, myasthenia gravis.
* Combination of both crises is often clinically encountered.

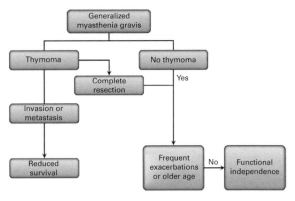

FIGURE 43.7: Outcome algorithm in myasthenia gravis. Functional independence: No assistance needed, minor handicap may remain.

Part VIII Postoperative Neurosurgical and Neurointerventional Complications

Chapter 44

Complications of Craniotomy and Biopsy

PRACTICAL NOTES

- A typical postcraniotomy order should include pain management with codeine, cefazolin, dexamethasone, phenytoin, and subcutaneous heparin; swallowing precautions; adequate fluids with crystalloids; and reduction of free water intake.
- Worsening after craniotomy may be due to hemorrhage in the surgical bed, remote hemorrhage, cerebral edema, or ischemic stroke from sacrifice of a large vein or artery.
- Careful evaluation of the endocrine axis (triiodothyronine, thyrotropin, cortisol, urine osmolarity) after pituitary surgery may detect panhypopituitarism.

TABLE 44.1. EXAMPLE OF A STANDARD POSTOPERATIVE CRANIOTOMY ORDER*

Codeine	30–60 mg IM, q4h p.r.n.
Cefazolin	1,000 mg IV, q8h
Dexamethasone	4 mg IV, q6h
Levetiracetam	1000 mg PO/IV, b.i.d.
Subcutaneous heparin	5,000 U, q8h

*Also includes swallowing precautions, incentive spirometry, crystalloid fluids, restriction of free water intake and continued treatment of increased intracranial pressure.

Chapter 45

Complications of Carotid Endarterectomy and Stenting

PRACTICAL NOTES

- Adequate postoperative blood pressure control and discontinuation of anticoagulation may be justified in patients at high risk for intracerebral hematomas.
- Admission to the NICU is warranted to monitor for wound hematomas, hypertension, and cardiac stress.
- Reexploration may be needed in stroke occurring after carotid endarterectomy.
- Carotid stenting may be briefly associated with symptomatic hypotension and bradycardia and is treatable with vasopressors and atropine.

TABLE 45.1. CLINICAL FEATURES OF CRANIAL NERVE DEFICITS AFTER CAROTID ENDARTERECTOMY

Type	Symptoms	Mechanism	Permanent
Facial nerve (VII)	Mimics central VII Asymmetry of upper lip	Hyperextension Head rotation	Rare
Glossopharyngeal nerve (IX)	Dysphagia Nasal regurgitation Hemiparesis Reduced soft palate constriction Hypertension common (Hering nerve)	Shunt placement (more retraction) Subluxation of mandible	Up to 5%

Vagus nerve (X)	Hoarseness Reduced coughing Inability to produce high tones	Ligation or transection of superior thyroid artery	Infrequent after 3 months
Accessory nerve (XI)	Drooping shoulder Painful acromioclavicular joint	Retractor injury Electrical trauma	Unclear
Hypoglossal nerve (XII)	Deviation of tongue Dysarthria Chewing difficulties	Short neck after transection of digastric muscle	Infrequent after 6 months

TABLE 45.2. TREATMENT FOR HYPOTENSION AND BRADYCARDIA AFTER CAROTID ARTERY STENTING

Atropine 0.5 mg with bradycardia

Fluid bolus 500 ml 0.9% NaCl

Phenylephrine bolus 200 mcg (repeat as needed or start 0.5 mcg/kg/minute infusion)

Keep MAP > 80 mm Hg

May start midodrine 10 mg t.i.d. before weaning phenylephrine

Adapted from Bujak et al. Dysautonomic responses during percutaneous carotid intervention: principles of physiology and management. *Catheter Cardiovasc Interv* 2015;85:282–291.

Chapter 46

Complications of Interventional Neuroradiology

PRACTICAL NOTES

- Most complications of interventional radiologic procedures are uncommon and usually manageable.
- Abciximab, intra-arterial thrombolysis, or mechanical disruption are good options in acute procedure-related emboli.
- Pericoil edema in endovascular treated aneurysms may be a cause of neurologic deterioration.

TABLE 46.1. PERINEUROINTERVENTIONAL MONITORING

Preinterventional evaluation

Concern for contrast medium allergy: methylprednisolone 80 mg IV or dexamethasone 16 mg IV 30 minutes
before procedure, in combination with promethazine 12.5 mg IV (over 1 minute), ranitidine 100 mg IV, and
montelukast sodium 10 mg PO

Concern for contrast-induced nephropathy: sodium bicarbonate 150 mEg/L IV solution at 3.5 ml/kg bolus over
1 hour, then 1.2 mL/kg/hr during procedure and for 6 hours after the procedure. *N*-acetylcysteine 600 mg
orally at 24 hours and 12 hours before and after the procedure (total of 4 doses)

Platelet count, international normalized ratio

Consult anesthesia for monitored sedation or full anesthesia

Postinterventional monitoring

Completely immobilize the accessed leg for several hours

Maintain SAP at ≤ 140 mm Hg (24 hours)

Avoid use of heparin or LMWH

Perform a follow-up computed tomographic scan of the brain at 12 hours

IV, intravenous; LMWH, low-molecular-weight heparin; PO, by mouth; SAP, systolic arterial pressure

Part IX Emergency Consults in the General Intensive Care Unit

Chapter 47

Neurology of Transplant Medicine

PRACTICAL NOTES

- CNS infections can be grouped in 6-month time periods and each has specific risks for certain organisms.
- Comatose patients with fulminant hepatic failure need ICP control before, during and after liver transplantation.
- Hematopoietic cell transplantation recipients have a high proclivity of drug neurotoxicity.
- Late neurologic complications may include CNS lymphoma or PML.

TABLE 47.1. CALCULATION
OF BRAIN EDEMA SEVERITY SCORE
(BESS), BASED ON COMPUTED
TOMOGRAPHIC FINDINGS IN PATIENTS
WITH FULMINANT HEPATIC FAILURE

Visibility of cortical sulci	
Visibility of cortical sulci	
3 CT scan slices of upper cerebral area (L/R)	6
Visibility of white matter	
Internal capsule (L/R)	2
Centrum semiovale (L/R)	2
Vertex (L/R)	2
Visibility of basal cisterns	
Sylvian fissure (horizontal-vertical, L/R)	4
Frontal interhemispheric fissure	1
Quadrigeminal cistern	1
Paired suprasellar cisterns (L/R)	2
Ambient cistern (L/R)	2
Maximal total BESS	22

CT, computed tomographic; L/R, left and right cerebral
hemispheres.
From Wijdicks EFM, Plevak DJ, Rakela J, Wiesner RH. Clinical and
radiologic features of cerebral edema in fulminant hepatic failure.
Mayo Clin Proc 1995;70:119–124.

TABLE 47.2. TREATMENT OPTIONS
OF BRAIN EDEMA IN FULMINANT
HEPATIC FAILURE

Hemodiafiltration to reduce serum ammonia to less
than 60 micromol/L

Moderate hypothermia (33°–35°C) with cooling
device and control of shivering

Propofol infusion (start with 30 mcg/kg per minute
and may increase to 200 mcg/kg per minute for
brief periods of time)

Mannitol, 0.5–1 g/kg every 6 hr if plasma osmolality
is < 310 mOsm/L

Hypertonic saline bolus (10%–23%) to serum
sodium of 150–155 mmol/L

Chapter 48

Neurology of Cardiac and Aortic Surgery

PRACTICAL NOTES

- Neurologic complications of cardiac and vascular surgery are not rare and remain an important cause of morbidity and mortality.
- Best evaluation of these complications requires a stat consult by the cardiac team.
- Spinal cord injury may be successfully treated with CSF diversion but only if MRI is normal.

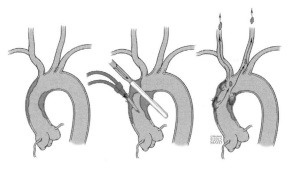

FIGURE 48.1: Ischemic stroke is likely caused by embolization out of damaged intravascular areas. Damage may be caused by clamping or catheter placement into severe atherosclerotic plaque.

TABLE 48.1. MANAGEMENT
OF POSTOPERATIVE STROKE
FOLLOWING CARDIAC SURGERY

Ischemic	Obtain CTA/CTP
	Endovascular retrieval if MCA M1/ M2 occlusion and large penumbra
	With large stroke avoid AC for 1–2 weeks
Hemorrhagic	Neurosurgical evacuation
	Correct INR with PCC
	Maintain INR < 1.3
	Platelet infusion if prior antiplatelet drugs
	Avoid antiplatelet agents
	Avoid AC for 1–2 weeks

CTA, computed tomography angiogram; CTP, computed tomography perfusion; M, middle cerebral artery; INR, international normalized ratio; AC, anticoagulation; PCC, prothrombin complex concentrate.

TABLE 48.2. INCIDENCE OF PARAPLEGIA

Crawford Classification	Incidence (Open Surgery)	Incidence (Endovascular)
I	7%	10%
II	24%	10%
III	22%	19%
IV	13%	5%
V	2%	3%

TABLE 48.3. ACUTE SPINAL CORD ISCHEMIA

CSF diversion (lumbar drainage)

Aim at ICP 8–12 mm Hg

Increase MAP 10 mm Hg every 5 minutes until improvement of MAP of 130 mm Hg reached

MRI spine for epidural hematoma or assessment for ischemia

Maintain MAP for 2 days and wean and remove lumbar drain

See references 10 and 11.

Chapter 49

Neurology of Resuscitation Medicine

PRACTICAL NOTES

- Repeat neurologic examination without confounders may identify poor outcome.
- MRI and SSEP are good (but not absolute) indicators of degree of injury.
- Therapeutic hypothermia is often associated with significant use of sedatives and analgesics, and clearance is poor.

TABLE 49.1. CLINICAL SYNDROMES
AFTER POSTANOXIC-ISCHEMIC
ENCEPHALOPATHY

Clinical Syndrome	Mechanism	Outcome
"Man-in-the-barrel" syndrome	Bilateral watershed infarcts	Uncertain, may improve substantially
Parkinsonism	Infarcts in the striatum	Improvement possible
Action myoclonus	Cerebellar infarcts	In awake patients, could improve with medication

TABLE 49.2. CONCERNS WHEN
EVALUATING PATIENTS TREATED
WITH HYPOTHERMIA

- Potentially confounded neurologic examination because hypothermia necessitates sedatives, neuromuscular blockers, and analgesics Motor response and corneal reflexes may not be reliable as early as day 3
- Decreased metabolism and clearance of sedative and analgesic medications related to hypothermia effects and kidney/liver injury
- Metabolic abnormalities and systemic shock
- Nonconvulsive seizures are possible during rewarming and require EEG for detection. Treatment is uncertain.

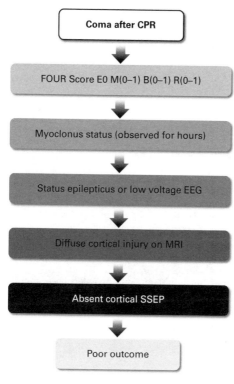

FIGURE 49.1: Framework for prognostication after CPR.

Chapter 50

Neurology of Pregnancy

PRACTICAL NOTES

- Endothelial dysfunction, hypersensitivity to angiotensin II resulting in acute hypertension, increased capillary permeability, and eventually brain edema are main components of eclampsia.
- Eclampsia does fall into the spectrum of posterior reversible encephalopathy syndrome and MRI images can be identical.
- Postpartum angiopathy may be reversible or rapidly fatal.

TABLE 50.1. FDA PREGNANCY RISK CATEGORIES

Category A	Controlled studies show no risk. Adequate, well-controlled studies in pregnant women have failed to demonstrate a risk to the fetus.
Category B	No evidence of risk in humans. Either animal study shows risk, but human findings do not, or if no adequate human studies have been done, animal findings are negative.
Category C	Risk cannot be ruled out. Human studies are lacking, and animal studies are either positive for fetal risk or lacking. However, potential benefits may justify potential risk.
Category D	Positive evidence of risk. Investigational or postmarketing data show risk to the fetus. Nevertheless, potential benefits may outweigh the potential risk.
Category X	Contraindicated in pregnancy. Studies in animals or humans or investigational or postmarketing reports have shown fetal risk, which clearly outweighs any possible benefit to the patient.
NA	FDA pregnancy category not available.

TABLE 50.2. ANTIEPILEPTIC DRUGS AND ASSOCIATED FETAL ANOMALIES

Antiepileptic drugs	Fetal anomalies
Carbamazepine	Neural tube defects, microcephaly, developmental delay, hypoplastic nails
Lamotrigine	Cleft lip, neural tube defects
Levetiracetam	Safety has not been established
Oxcarbazepine	Cleft lip, neural tube defects
Phenobarbital	Distal digital hypoplasia, low set ears, cleft lip, cleft palate, developmental delay, ptosis
Phenytoin	Cleft lip, cleft palate, heart malformations, and other minor birth defects (short fingers, widely spaced eyes)
Valproic acid	Neural tube defects, spina bifida, cleft lip, cleft palate, organ malformations, limb deficiencies, developmental delay

TABLE 50.3. MATERNAL CARDIAC ARREST (BEAU-CHOPS)

Bleeding/DIC
Embolism: coronary/pulmonary/amniotic fluid
  embolism
Anesthetic complications
Uterine atony
Cardiac disease (MI/ischemia/aortic dissection/
  cardiomyopathy)
Hypertension/preeclampsia/eclampsia
Other: differential diagnosis of standard ACLS
  guidelines
Placenta abruptio/previa
Sepsis

Adapted from reference 17

TABLE 50.4. MAJOR NEUROLOGIC DISORDERS OF PREGNANCY AND PUERPERUM

Eclampsia
Ischemic stroke
Lobar cerebral hematoma
Ruptured cerebral aneurysm or AVM
Postpartum angiopathy
Posterior reversible encephalopathy syndrome
Amniotic fluid embolism
Choriocarcinoma
Pituitary apoplexy
Thrombotic thrombocytopenic purpura
Glioma or other malignancy

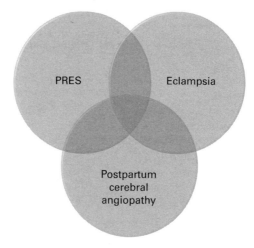

FIGURE 50.1: Overlap between posterior reversible enceph-alopathy syndrome (PRES), eclampsia, and angiopathy in pregnancy.

Part X Critical Care Support

Chapter 51

Shock

PRACTICAL NOTES

- The 4 major causes of shock are cardiac, vasodilatory, hypovolemic or obstructive causes.
- The initial management is a fluid challenge with normal saline but often norepinephrine are needed.
- Systolic blood pressure of at least 90 mm Hg must be maintained.
- Mechanical support is needed in cardiogenic shock if inotropes and vasopressors have a limited effect

TABLE 51.1. DEFINITIONS OF SYSTEMIC INFLAMMATORY RESPONSE SYNDROME (SIRS), SEPSIS, SEVERE SEPSIS, AND SEPTIC SHOCK

Term	Criteria
SIRS	Meets two of the following four:
	Temperature > 38°C or < 36°C
	Heart rate > 90 beats/min
	Respiratory rate > 30 breaths/min or arterial CO_2 < 32 mm Hg
	White blood cell count > 12,000 or < 4,000 cells/µL or >10% band forms
Sepsis	Documented or suspected infection plus systemic manifestations of infection (any of the SIRS criteria in addition other possible manifestations including elevations of procalcitonin, C-reactive protein, hyperglycemia in those without diabetes)
Severe sepsis	Sepsis plus evidence of organ dysfunction
	Arterial hypoxemia (PaO_2/FiO_2 < 300)
	Acute oliguria (urine output < 0.5 mL/kg per hour for at least 2 hours despite adequate fluid resuscitation)
	Increase in creatinine > 0.5 mg/dL
	Coagulation abnormalities (INR > 1.5, aPTT > 60 s, platelets < 100,000/µL)
	Hepatic dysfunction (elevated bilirubin)
	Paralytic ileus
	Decreased capillary refill or skin mottling
Septic shock	Sepsis with hypotension refractory to fluid resuscitation or hyperlactatemia
	Refractory hypotension persists despite resuscitation with bolus intravenous fluid of 30 mL/kg
	Hyperlactatemia > 2 mmol/L

aPTT, activated partial thromboplastin time; INR, international normalized ratio.

TABLE 51.2. COMMON VASOACTIVE DRUGS IN SHOCK

Vasopressor	Dose	Effect
Epinephrine	0.07–1 mcg/kg/min	↑ SVR
Norepinephrine	0.04–1 mcg/kg/min	↑ SVR
Phenylephrine	0.5–5 mcg/kg/min	↑ SVR
Vasopressin	0.04 U/min	↑ SVR
Dopamine	5–20 mcg/kg/min	↑ SVR, ↑ CI
Milrinone	0.375–0.75 mcg/kg/min	↑ CI

TABLE 51.3. THERAPEUTICS FOR ANAPHYLAXIS AFTER INTRAMUSCULAR EPINEPHRINE

Intervention	Dose and Route of Administration
Volume expansion	
0.9% saline	Adult: 1–2 L rapidly IV (5–10 ml/kg in first 5 min); child: 20 ml/kg in first hour
Epinephrine infusion	1 mg of 1:1,000 v/v (1 mg/ml) dilution added to 250 ml 5% dextrose in water (or NS) (i.e., 4 μg/ml concentration) infused at 1–4 μg/min (15–60 drops/min with microdrop), increasing to maximum 10 μg/min
Antihistamines	
Diphenhydramine	Adult: 25–50 mg IV; child: 1 mg/kg IV, up to 50 mg, infused over 10 min

(*continued*)

TABLE 51.3. (CONTINUED)

Corticosteroids

Methylprednisolone   1–2 mg/kg/day IV

Vasopressors

Dopamine	400 mg in 500 ml 5% dextrose in water infused at 2–5 µg/kg/min
Glucagon	Initial dose, 1–5 mg slow IV, then 5–15 µg/min infusion
Methylene blue	Single-bolus 1.5–2 mg/kg in 100 ml 5% dextrose in water infused over 20 min has been used

Adapted from Kemp AM, Kemp SF. Pharmacotherapy in refractory anaphylaxis: when intramuscular epinephrine fails. *Curr Opin Allergy Clin Immunol* 2014;14:371–378.

TABLE 51.4. SHOCK INDEX

SHOCK INDEX (SI) = *HR/SBP*	
No shock	SI < 0.6
Mild shock	SI 0.6–0.9
Moderate shock	SI 1.0–1.3
Severe shock	SI ≥ 1.4

TABLE 51.5. HEMORRHAGIC SHOCK

RESUSCITATION GOALS
SBP < 90 mm Hg
SPO2 > 96%
Hemoglobin 7–9 g/dL
Fibrinogen > 1.5g/L
INR ≤ 1.5
Platelets >50 g/L

From reference 12.

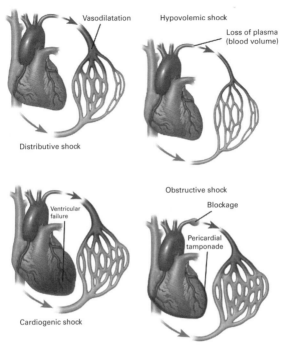

FIGURE 51.1: Different shock states usually are defined by cardiac function and state of peripheral circulation.

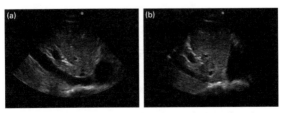

FIGURE 51.2: Ultrasound with subcostal view showing (A) normal IVC and (B) near 100% collapsibility.

Chapter 52

Cardiopulmonary arrest

PRACTICAL NOTES

- Important first decision is to start chest compression and ventilation (compression/ventilation 30:2 ratio).
- Important second decision is to determine rhythm and whether shockable
- Important third decision is to treat remaining cardiac arrhythmia
- Low end-tidal CO_2, prolonged effort in asystole, and absent brainstem reflexes in a normothermic patient may indicate failure of CPR.

TABLE 52.2. POST–CARDIAC ARREST SYNDROME: PATHOPHYSIOLOGY, CLINICAL MANIFESTATIONS, AND POTENTIAL TREATMENTS

Syndrome	Pathophysiology	Clinical Manifestation	Potential Treatments
Post–cardiac arrest myocardial dysfunction	Global hypokinesis (myocardial stunning) ACS	Reduced cardiac output Hypotension Dysrhythmias Cardiovascular collapse	Early revascularization of AMI Early hemodynamic optimization Intravenous fluid Inotropes IABP LVAD ECMO
Systemic ischemia/ reperfusion response	Systemic inflammatory response syndrome Impaired vasoregulation Increased coagulation Adrenal suppression Impaired tissue oxygen delivery and utilization Impaired resistance to infection	Ongoing tissue hypoxia/ ischemia Hypotension Cardiovascular collapse Pyrexia (fever) Hyperglycemia Multiorgan failure Infection	Early hemodynamic optimization IV fluid Vasopressors High-volume hemofiltration Temperature control Glucose control Antibiotics with documented infection

ACS indicates acute coronary syndrome; AMI, acute myocardial infarction; ECMO, extracorporeal membrane oxygenation; IABP, intra-aortic balloon pump; IV, intravenous; LVAD, left ventricular assist device.
Adapted from Neumar et al. Post-cardiac arrest syndrome: epidemiology, pathophysiology, treatment, and prognostication. *Circulation* 2008;118:2452–2483. Copyright ©2008, American Heart Association, Inc.

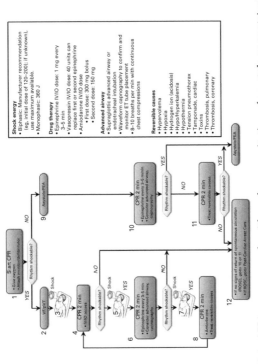

FIGURE 52.1: AHA consensus algorithms for resuscitation of asystole or ventricular fibrillation (copyright sign American Heart Association).

Chapter 53

Acute Kidney Injury

PRACTICAL NOTES

- Acute renal failure in the NICU is often related to hypotension, newly introduced antibiotics and as a result of rhabdomyolysis.
- Contrast-induced nephropathy can be prevented with fluid therapy alone
- Renal replacement therapy should be considered in patients with anuria, elevated potassium and evidence of fluid overload
- Renal replacement therapy (either intermittent or continuous) may leads to dialysis disequilibrium syndrome and consequently increases ICP but less with continuous mode

TABLE 53.1. RIFLE CRITERIA

	Creatinine	Urinary Output
Risk	Increase creatinine × 1.5 or acute rise ≥ 0.3 mg/dL	UO < 0.5 mL/kg/hr for 6 hours
Injury	Increased creatinine × 2	UO < 0.5 mL/kg/hr for 12 hours
Failure	Increased creatinine × 3 or creatinine > 4 mg/dL	UO < 0.3 mL/kg/hr for 24 hours or anuria for 12 hours
Loss		Complete loss of function > 4 weeks
ESRD	End-stage	Renal disease dialysis dependent

TABLE 53.2. COMMON CAUSES OF ACUTE KIDNEY INJURY IN THE NICU

Acute blood loss in polytrauma
Drug induced hypotension
Hypovolemia
Vancomycin, acyclovir, NSAIDs
Rhabdomyolysis
Sepsis
Recent major surgery
Contrast dye

TABLE 53.3. CLINICAL MANIFESTATIONS ASSOCIATED WITH ACUTE KIDNEY INJURY

Complication	Clinical Manifestation
Hyponatremia	Abnormal mentation and seizure
Hyperkalemia	Cardiac arrhythmias (including malignant types)
Volume overload	Pulmonary edema
	Pulmonary hemorrhage
	Acute hypertension
	Abdominal compartment syndrome
Anemia and thrombocythemia	Hemorrhage
Anion gap metabolic Acidosis	Cardiorespiratory abnormalities
Gut ischemia	Acute gastrointestinal hemorrhage
Uremia	Stupor, coma

TABLE 53.4. DRUGS THAT REQUIRE
DECREASE OR AVOIDANCE IN ACUTE
RENAL FAILURE

Drug	Adjustment with CLCR < 60 mL/min
Codeine	Up to 50%
Midazolam	Up to 50%
Acyclovir	Increase dosing interval or decrease 25%
Cephalosporins	Decrease
Vancomycin	Monitor serum level and adjust
Phenytoin	Monitor free drug level

TABLE 53.5. CRITERIA FOR THE
INITIATION OF RENAL REPLACEMENT
THERAPY (RRT) IN THE ICU

Anuria (no urine output for 6 hours)
Oliguria (urine output < 200 mL/12 hours)
BUN > 80 mg/dL or urea > 28 mmol/L
Creatinine > 3 mg/L or > 265 μmol/L
Serum potassium > 6.5 mmol/L or rapidly rising
Pulmonary edema unresponsive to diuretics
Uncompensated metabolic acidosis (pH < 7.1)
Uremic complications (encephalopathy/myopathy/
neuropathy/pericarditis)

If one criterion is present, RRT should be considered. If two criteria
are simultaneously present, RRT is strongly recommended.

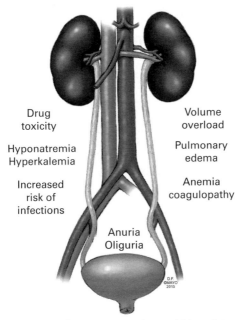

Drug
toxicity

Hyponatremia
Hyperkalemia

Increased
risk of
infections

Volume
overload

Pulmonary
edema

Anemia
coagulopathy

Anuria
Oliguria

D.F.
©MAYO
2015

FIGURE 53.2: Consequences of acute kidney injury in the NICU.

Chapter 54

Endocrine Emergencies

PRACTICAL NOTES

- Treatment of both DKA and HHS is adequate fluid administration with isotonic saline and correction of potassium deficit.
- Major thyroid abnormalities may lead to impaired consciousness with good response to replacement of T3 or blocking with propylthiouracil.
- Unexpected hypothermia and bradycardia may indicate severe hypothyroidism.
- Initially, most patients with pituitary apoplexy are not urgent surgical candidates and not in endocrine crises but may worsen quickly.

TABLE 54.1. LABORATORY CRITERIA DIABETIC KETOACIDOSIS (DKA) AND HYPERGLYCEMIC HYPEROSMOLAR COMA (HHC)

Laboratory	DKA	HHC
Blood glucose	> 250 mg/dL	> 600 mg/dL
Arterial blood gas	pH < 7.3	pH > 7.3
	Bicarb < 18	Bicarb > 18
Anion gap	Increased	Mostly normal
Plasma osmolality	Normal to increased	Increased
Ketones in urine	++	±

Data from Keays R. Diabetic emergencies. In: Oh TE, Soni N, eds. *Oh's Intensive Care Manual*. 5th ed. Oxford: Butterworth-Heinemann, 2003; Kitabchi AE, Umpierrez GE, Murphy MB, et al. Hyperglycemic crises in patients with diabetes mellitus. *Diabetes Care* 2003;26 Suppl 1:S109–S117; Maletkovic J, Drexler A. Diabetic ketoacidosis and hyperglycemic hyperosmolar state. *Endocrinol Metab Clin N Am* 2013;42:677–695.

TABLE 54.2. PRECIPITATING FACTORS IN MYXEDEMATOUS COMA

General anesthesia
Narcotics
Sedatives
Amiodarone
Lithium carbonate
Infection
Hypothermia (incidental)

TABLE 54.3. PRESENTING SIGNS
OF PITUITARY APOPLEXY
(IN ORDER OF FREQUENCY)

Thunderclap (or acute) headache
Nausea and vomiting
Visual field defect
Third-nerve palsy
Sixth-nerve palsy
Multiple cranial nerve palsies
Facial pain

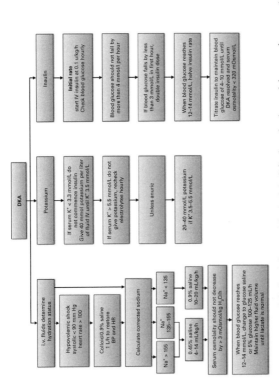

FIGURE 54.1: Management of diabetic ketoacidosis. Modified and adapted from references 14, 17, 18

Part XI Management of Systemic Complications

Chapter 55

Management of Pulmonary Complications

PRACTICAL NOTES

- The most common cause of acute hypoxemic respiratory failure in the NICU is ventilation–perfusion mismatch from atelectasis, aspiration, pulmonary edema, or pulmonary embolism.
- Sudden respiratory distress in a mechanically ventilated patient should prompt disconnection (to demonstrate machine failure), tracheal suctioning or bronchoscopy (to demonstrate bronchial obstruction), chest radiography (to demonstrate pulmonary infiltrates or pneumothorax), and helical CT scan (to demonstrate pulmonary emboli). Inappropriate ventilator settings may cause patient–ventilator asynchrony.

TABLE 55.1. INITIAL BEDSIDE APPROACH TO ACUTE HYPOXEMIC RESPIRATORY FAILURE

A–a Gradient	Other Variable	Disorder
Normal	PI_{max} decreased	Neuromuscular cause of hypoventilation
	PI_{max} normal	Central cause of hypoventilation
Increased	Correction with 100% O_2	Ventilation–perfusion mismatch
	No correction with 100% O_2	Right-to-left shunt, intraparenchymal or intracardiac

A–a, alveolar-arterial; PI_{max}, maximum inspiratory pressure.

TABLE 55.2. INITIAL BEDSIDE APPROACH TO ACUTE HYPERCAPNIC RESPIRATORY FAILURE

A–a Gradient	Other Variable	Disorder
Normal	PI_{max} decreased	Neuromuscular
	PI_{max} normal	
	Increased CO_2 production	Sepsis, seizures
	Normal CO_2 production	Central hypoventilation
Increased		Cardiopulmonary

A–a, alveolar-arterial; PI_{max}, maximum inspiratory pressure.

TABLE 55.3. DIFFERENTIAL DIAGNOSIS OF ACUTE RESPIRATORY DISTRESS IN MECHANICALLY VENTILATED PATIENTS

Acute main bronchus obstruction
Pneumothorax
Atelectasis
Pulmonary embolus
Pulmonary edema
Dislodgment of tracheostomy
Endotracheal malposition
Inappropriate ventilator setting
Ventilator dysfunction
Abdominal distention

TABLE 55.4. LABORATORY TEST RESULTS SUPPORTIVE OF PULMONARY EMBOLISM AND INCREASING THE PROBABILITY OF A DIAGNOSTIC HELICAL CT OF THE CHEST

Hypocapnia and hypoxemia
Electrocardiographic abnormalities
T-wave inversion in the right precordial leads, III, and aVF
ST depression (nonreciprocal)
T-wave inversion (patients with history of cardiopulmonary disease)
Sudden atrial fibrillation
P pulmonale
Right bundle-branch block
D-dimer increase (> 500 μg/L)
Increased right ventricular dimension or dilated right pulmonary artery on echocardiography

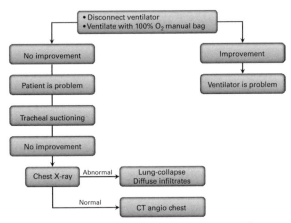

FIGURE 55.1: Algorithm for initial management of mechanically ventilated patients in acute respiratory distress.

Chapter 56

Management of Cardiac Complications

PRACTICAL NOTES

- Most cardiac arrhythmias in acute CNS disorders are transient and do not require therapeutic intervention.
- Atrial fibrillation with rapid ventricular rate is common in patients admitted to the NICU and responds well to IV diltiazem.
- The most common morphologic EKG changes in acute CNS catastrophes are prolonged QT interval, ST segment sagging, and deeply inverted T waves. They may be difficult to distinguish from patterns seen in acute myocardial infarction.
- Echocardiography may be a useful noninvasive tool for early diagnosis of cardiac anatomical or functional abnormalities that may underlie the arrhythmias.
- The risk of cardiac mortality and nonfatal myocardial infarction with craniotomy is less than 5% but increases in patients with unstable angina, congestive heart failure, cardiac arrhythmias, or valvular disease.

TABLE 56.1. ELECTROCARDIOGRAPHIC CHANGES IN SUBARACHNOID HEMORRHAGE*

	No. of Patients
Ischemic ST segment	44
Ischemic T wave	41
Prominent U wave	39
QT$_c$ interval prolongation	34
Flat or isoelectric T wave	24
Short PR interval	14
Long PR interval	13
Transient pathologic Q wave	11
Peaked P wave	10
Tall T wave	10
Broad P wave	4

*Based on findings in 61 patients with serial electrocardiograms.
Modified from Brouwers PJ, Wijdicks EFM, Hasan D, et al. Serial electrocardiographic recording in aneurysmal subarachnoid hemorrhage. *Stroke* 1989;20:1162–1167. With permission of the American Heart Association.

TABLE 56.2. INTRAVENOUS ANTIARRHYTHMIC DRUGS

Drug	Dose	Side Effects
Atropine	0.5–1.0 mg as a rapid bolus, max 3 mg	Sinus tachycardia
Adenosine	6 mg in 2 minutes; if no effect, 12 mg	Profound hypotension, facial flushing, bradycardia
Diltiazem	0.25 mg/kg (actual body weight) bolus over 2 minutes; maintenance 5–15 mg per hour	Hypotension, heart block, headache
Verapamil	5–10 mg bolus over 3 minutes; repeated if necessary may be followed by continuous infusion of 0.005 mg/kg per minute	Headache, nausea, constipation, hypotension, heart block
Lidocaine	0.7–1.4 mg/kg bolus over 3 minutes followed by 1–4 mg/minute constant infusion	Seizures, respiratory arrest, dizziness, heart block (usually associated with preexisting abnormal His-Purkinje conduction), sinoatrial arrest
Procainamide	100 mg IV slowly (25 mg/minute) to maximum 1,000 mg	Hypotension, prolonged AV and His-Purkinje conduction

(continued)

TABLE 56.2. (CONTINUED)

Drug	Dose	Side Effects
Metoprolol	5 mg every 5 minutes up to 15 mg	Hypotension, bradycardia, prolonged AV conduction and heart block, myocardial depression
Propranolol	1 mg/minute every 5 minutes up to 10 mg	Hypotension, bradycardia, prolonged AV conduction and heart block, myocardial depression, bronchospasm
Esmolol	0.5 mg/kg bolus, 0.05–0.2 mg/kg per minute infusion	Hypotension, bradycardia, bronchoconstriction
Magnesium sulfate	1 g in 10 mL of normal saline over 20 minutes or 1–4 g/hour infusion	Diarrhea, flushing

AV, atrioventricular; IV, intravenously.

TABLE 56.3. GUIDELINES FOR THE INITIAL MANAGEMENT OF COMMON CARDIAC ARRHYTHMIAS

Arrhythmia	Therapy
Sinus tachycardia	Esmolol
Sinus bradycardia	Atropine, cardiac pacing
Atrial fibrillation (RVR)	Diltiazem, verapamil
Atrial flutter (RVR)	Diltiazem, verapamil
Multifocal atrial tachycardia	Verapamil or metoprolol
Junctional rhythm	Atropine
Atrioventricular block	Cardiac pacing
Ventricular tachycardia	Cardioversion
Torsades de pointes	Magnesium sulfate

RVR, rapid ventricular response.

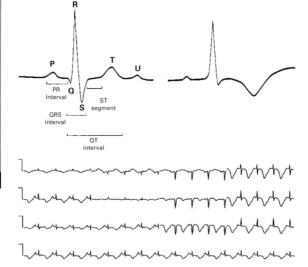

FIGURE 56.1: Typical morphologic changes in electrocardiographic tracing associated with acute severe brain injury. Note these changes in EKG. *Left*: Normal tracing. *Right*: Abnormal tracing with ST-segment depression, marked T-wave inversion, and QT interval prolongation.

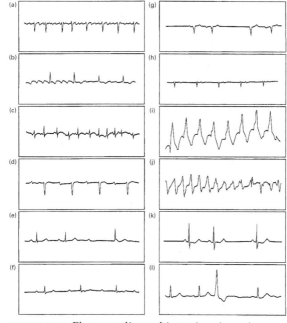

FIGURE 56.5: Electrocardiographic tracings in various arrhythmias. (A) Atrial fibrillation. (B) Atrial flutter. (C) Multifocal atrial tachycardia. (D) Junctional rhythm. (E) First-degree atrioventricular block. (F) Second-degree atrioventricular block (Mobitz type I). (G) Second-degree atrioventricular block (Mobitz type II). (H) Third-degree atrioventricular block. (I) Ventricular tachycardia. (J) Torsades de pointes. (K) Premature atrial complex. (L) Premature ventricular complex.

Chapter 57

Management of Acid–Base Disorders, Sodium and Glucose Handling

PRACTICAL NOTES

- Most patients with metabolic acidosis in the NICU have transient lactic acidosis after seizures. A major systemic illness should be considered in other circumstances.
- Hyponatremia must be viewed against volume status. Cerebral salt wasting (hypovolemic hyponatremia) is more common in certain CNS disorders than SIADH (normovolemic hyponatremia). The laboratory criteria are virtually identical. Differentiation from SIADH is possible with serial body weight (decrease), fluid balance (negative), and with clinical signs of early dehydration, relative tachycardia, orthostasis, and marginal skin turgor.
- Hypernatremia from dehydration is most common with diabetes insipidus from traumatic brain injury, at the time of diagnosis of brain death, or with use of osmotic diuretic agents.
- Hyperglycemia is a stress response after any major acute neurologic illness. Treatment of severe hyperglycemia is warranted, aiming at glucose values between 140 and 180 mg/dL. These target levels may need revision in the future.

TABLE 57.1. REPLACEMENT THERAPY IN ELECTROLYTE ABNORMALITIES OTHER THAN SODIUM DISORDER

Electrolyte Abnormality	Cause	Consequences	Treatment*
Hypomagnesemia	Gastrointestinal and renal loss, drug interaction	Cardiac arrhythmias, muscle weakness	1–2 g of magnesium sulfate in 20 mL of normal saline over 5–20 minutes
Hypermagnesemia	Renal failure, antacids, enemas	Muscle weakness, hypotension, asystole	1–2 grams of calcium gluconate IV over 15 minutes
Hypercalcemia	Diabetes insipidus, malignancy, hyper-parathyroidism	Seizures, coma, cardiac arrhythmias	Hydration, 0.9% NaCl, 500 mL/hour
Hypocalcemia	Critical illness, hypoparathyroidism, fat-deficient diet	Cardiac arrhythmias, tetanus, seizures, laryngospasm	1–2 g of calcium gluconate IV over 15 minutes; then 6 g of calcium gluconate in 500 mL normal saline with infusion for 4–6 hours

(continued)

TABLE 57.1. (CONTINUED)

Electrolyte Abnormality	Cause	Consequences	Treatment*
Hypophosphatemia	Parenteral nutrition, preexisting alcoholism, renal failure	Congestive cardiomyopathy, respiratory failure, rhabdomyolysis	Potassium phosphate, 0.08 mmol/kg IV in 500 mL of 0.45% saline over 6 hours
Hyperphosphatemia	Rare	Similar to those with hypocalcemia	Phosphate binders, 1 g of calcium PO t.i.d.
Hypokalemia	Vomiting, prolonged starvation, gastrointestinal loss	Ventricular fibrillation, quadriplegia	KCL 10 mEq/hour IV infusion
Hyperkalemia	Crush injury, hemolysis, renal failure	Cardiac arrest	1 gram of calcium gluconate IV over 5 minutes

IV, intravenously.
*When markedly abnormal.
Data from Singer GG. Fluid and electrolyte management. In Ahya SN, Flood K, Paranjothi S, eds. *Washington Manual of Medical Therapeutics.* 30th ed. Philadelphia: Lippincott Williams & Wilkins; 2001: 43–75. With permission of the publisher.

TABLE 57.2. COMMON CAUSES
OF METABOLIC ACIDOSIS IN THE NICU

Lactic acidosis (status epilepticus)
Ketoacidosis (diabetes, alcoholism, malnourishment)
Septic shock
Rhabdomyolysis
Diarrhea
Hyperalimentation

TABLE 57.3. COMMON CAUSES
OF METABOLIC ALKALOSIS IN THE NICU

Excessive vomiting
Gastrointestinal losses
Diuretics (loop or thiazide)
Massive blood transfusion in multitrauma
Severe hypokalemia
Sodium bicarbonate infusion

TABLE 57.4. COMMON CAUSES OF
RESPIRATORY ACIDOSIS IN THE NICU

Aspiration pneumonitis
Adult respiratory distress syndrome
Acute pulmonary edema
Pneumothorax
Neuromuscular respiratory failure (end stage)

TABLE 57.5. COMMON CAUSES
OF RESPIRATORY ALKALOSIS
IN THE NICU

Induced hyperventilation
Mechanical ventilation
Intracranial pressure management
Compensatory response to hypoxemia
Adult respiratory distress syndrome
Pulmonary embolism
Central neurogenic hyperventilation
Early sepsis
Postoperative pain and anxiety

TABLE 57.6. POTENTIAL CAUSES
OF HYPO-OSMOLAR HYPONATREMIA
IN THE NICU

Hypovolemia	Normovolemia or Hypervolemia
Diuretics (thiazide, loop)	SIADH
Addison's disease (acute corticosteroid withdrawal)	Acute renal failure
	Congestive heart failure
Gastrointestinal and skin losses	
Dietary sodium restriction (with excess hypotonic fluid intake)	Hepatic failure
Cerebral salt wasting	

SIADH, syndrome of inappropriate antidiuretic hormone.

TABLE 57.7. TREATMENT OF SYMPTOMATIC HYPONATREMIA

Volume Contraction	Volume Dilution
0.9% NaCl (or 1.5%)	Calculate need to normalize serum sodium by using
3% NaCl*	3% NaCl (513 mmol/L) in the formula
Fludrocortisone acetate, 0.4 mg/day	$\dfrac{513 - \text{current serum Na}}{0.5 \times \text{body weight (kg)} + 1}$
	to provide total millimoles per liter
	Rate: raise serum sodium 1 mmol/L/hr

*Patient needs a central venous catheter placed.
A calculator is available on www.medcalc.com.
Data from Adrogué HJ, Madias NE. Hyponatremia. *N Engl J Med* 2000;342:1581–1589. With permission of the Massachusetts Medical Society.

TABLE 57.8. CAUSES OF HYPERNATREMIA IN THE NICU

Hypovolemia	Normovolemia or Hypervolemia
Gastrointestinal loss	Hypertonic sodium solutions
Diuretics (e.g., mannitol)	Corticosteroid excess
Diabetes insipidus	
Increased insensible fluid loss	

TABLE 57.9. TREATMENT
OF SYMPTOMATIC HYPERNATREMIA

Pure Water Loss or Hypotonic Hypernatremic	Hypertonic Hypernatremia
Calculate need to normalize serum sodium by using 5% dextrose in the formula:	Furosemide, 40–80 mg IV; switch to electrolyte-free water infusion (5% dextrose)

$$\frac{0 - \text{current plasma Na}}{0.5 \times \text{body weight} + 1}$$

Or

0.45% NaCl in the formula:

$$\frac{77 - \text{current plasma Na}}{0.5 \times \text{body weight} + 1}$$

to provide total millimoles
per liter
Rate: reduce serum sodium
10 mmol/L in 24 hours
Desmopressin, 2–4 mcg IV
in 2 divided doses

A calculator is available on www.medcalc.com
Data from Adrogué HJ, Madias NE. Hypernatremia. *N Engl J Med* 2000;342:1493–1499. With permission of the Massachusetts Medical Society.

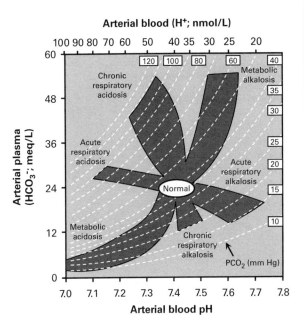

FIGURE 57.1: Acid–base nomogram. Boxed values are arterial PCO_2.

Modified from DuBose TD Jr. Acid-base disorders. In Brenner BM, ed., *Brenner & Rector's The Kidney,* 6th ed. Vol. 1. Philadelphia: W. B. Saunders, 2000: 925–997. With permission of the publisher.

Chapter 58

Management of Gastrointestinal Complications

PRACTICAL NOTES

- The severity of gastrointestinal hemorrhage should be assessed immediately. Potentially ominous clinical signs are orthostatic hypotension and tachycardia with change in position. Tachycardia with position change but without change in blood pressure indicates a 15% loss of volume, and decrease in blood pressure to 100 mm Hg with position change indicates a 25% or greater volume loss.
- Endoscopy is indicated in patients with gastrointestinal bleeding and need for transfusion.
- Management in gastrointestinal hemorrhage is focused on volume resuscitation and preservation of adequate blood pressure. Proton-pump inhibitors should be administered early.
- Diarrhea is most commonly associated with enteral nutrition and release of fecal impaction related to narcotic analgesics or dehydration.
- Adynamic ileus is usually treated with oral and rectal tubes, no oral intake, and intravenous neostigmine.
- Traumatic abdominal injury may be subtle, and CT scanning and repeat examination for abdominal tenderness are needed within the first day of admission. Laparotomy is required in hemodynamically unstable patients.

TABLE 58.1. MANAGEMENT OF ACUTE
UPPER GASTROINTESTINAL BLEEDING

Mallory-Weiss syndrome	Volume resuscitation
	Endoscopic confirmation
	Observation or electrocoagulation
Peptic ulcer, erosions	Volume resuscitation
	Endoscopic confirmation
	Proton-pump inhibitors
	Surgery if at increased risk for rebleeding

TABLE 58.2. CAUSES OF DIARRHEA
IN NICU

Hyperosmolar enteral nutrition
Enteral feeding at high infusion rates
Antacids, clindamycin, cephalosporins, histamine$_2$-receptor antagonists, angiotensin-converting enzyme inhibitors, theophylline
Hypoalbuminemia
Clostridium difficile infection

TABLE 58.3. POSSIBLE CAUSES
OF PARALYTIC ILEUS AND OGILVIE
SYNDROME

Neurologic disorders
Guillain-Barré syndrome
Meningitis
Spinal cord injury
Surgical procedures
Abdominal exploration for blunt trauma and shock
Drugs
Opioids
Tricyclic antidepressants
Phenothiazines

See also Vanek VW, Al-Salti M. Acute pseudo-obstruction of the colon (Ogilvie's syndrome): an analysis of 400 cases. *Dis Colon Rectum* 1986;29:203–210.

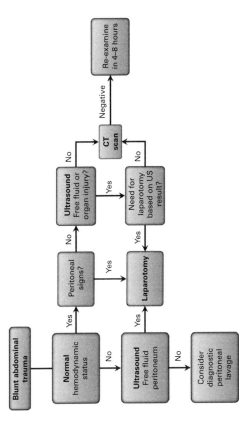

FIGURE 58.5: Algorithm for abdominal trauma.

CT, computed tomography; US, ultrasound.

Modified from Amoroso TA. Evaluation of the patient with blunt abdominal trauma: an evidence based approach. *Emerg Med Clin N Am* 1999;17:63–75. With permission of W. B. Saunders Company.

Chapter 59

Management of Nosocomial Infections

PRACTICAL NOTES

- New-onset fever often indicates infection but may be caused by resorption of blood (relative bradycardia), thromboembolism (persistent tachycardia, painful calves), or drugs (incremental increase in temperature within several days).
- Nosocomial pneumonia is typically recognized by fever, peripheral infiltrates on chest radiographs, change in sputum quality to purulent mucus, and ≥25 polymorphonuclear leukocytes on Gram's stain.
- Phlebitis remains the most common catheter-related infection. Changing the catheter site and applying cold, wet compresses are often sufficient. Catheter-associated bacteremia is an emergency that should be treated by intravenous administration of vancomycin and a cephalosporin.
- Nosocomial urinary tract infections in catheterized patients are diagnosed by increased leukocyte counts (>10 cells/mm^3) and cultures. When gram-positive cocci are suspected, vancomycin is preferred.
- Nosocomial gastrointestinal infections are invariably caused by *C. difficile*. Metronidazole is given orally.
- Ventriculitis can be effectively treated with vancomycin and cefotaxime intravenously, assuming that *S. epidermidis* and *aureus* are the causative agents.

TABLE 59.1. COMMONLY FOUND
ORGANISMS IN ASPIRATION
PNEUMONIA

Community acquired	Healthcare acquired
Haemophilus influenzae	Anaerobes *Streptococcus*
Streptococcus pneumonia	Other otopharyngeal
Anaerobes	*Streptococcus aureus*
Other otopharyngeal	*Enterobacteriaceae*
Streptococcus	*Pseudomonas aeruginosa*

TABLE 59.2. THE MODIFIED PULMONARY INFECTION SCORE

CPIS Points	0	1	2
Tracheal secretions	Rare	Abundant	Abundant + purulent
Chest X-ray infiltrates	No infiltrate	Diffuse	Localized
Temperature, °C	≥ 36.5 and ≤ 38.4	≥ 38.5 and ≤ 38.9	≥ 39 or ≤ 36
Leukocytes count, per mm^3	$\geq 4,000$ and $\leq 11,000$	$< 4,000$ or $> 11,000$	$< 4,000$ or $> 11,000$ + band forms $\geq 50\%$
PaO$_2$/FIO$_2$ mm Hg	> 240 or ARDS		≤ 240 and no evidence of ARDS
Microbiology	Negative		Positive

Definitions of abbreviations: ARDS, acute respiratory distress syndrome; CPIS, clinical pulmonary infection score. The modified CPIS at baseline was calculated from the first five variables. The CPIS Gram and CPIS culture were calculated from the CPIS baseline score by adding two more points when Gram stains or culture were positive. A score of more than 6 at baseline or after incorporating the Gram stains (CPIS gram) or culture (CPIS culture) results was considered suggestive of pneumonia. Fartoukh M, Maitre B, Honoré S, et al. Diagnosing pneumonia during mechanical ventilation: the Clinical Pulmonary Infection Score revisited. *Am J Respir Crit Care Med* 2003;168:173–179.

TABLE 59.3. INITIAL ANTIMICROBIAL
TREATMENT FOR HOSPITAL-ACQUIRED
OR VENTILATOR-ASSOCIATED
PNEUMONIA

Antipseudomonal cephalosporin	
Cefepime	1–2 gram every 8–12 hours
Ceftazidime	2 gram every 8 hours
or	
β-lactam/β-lactamase inhibitor	
Piperacillin/tazobactam plus	4.5 gram every 6 hours
Antipseudomonal fluoroquinolone	
Ciprofloxacin	400 mg every 8 hours
Levofloxacin	750 mg every day

TABLE 59.4. ANTIMICROBIAL
TREATMENT OF CATHETER-RELATED
BACTEREMIA OR SEPSIS

Vancomycin	15–20 mg/kg IV 12 h
with cefotaxime	1–2 g q6h IV
or	
Vancomycin	2 g q12h IV
with gentamicin	1.5–1.7 mg/kg q8h IV

TABLE 59.5. ANTIMICROBIAL TREATMENT OF NOSOCOMIAL URINARY TRACT INFECTION

Gentamicin	1–1.3 mg/kg q8h IV
or	
Ceftriaxone	1–2 g q24h IV
or	
Ciprofloxacin	0.2–0.4 g q12h IV
or	
Ampicillin	0.5 g q6h IV
with gentamicin	1 mg/kg q8h IV

TABLE 59.6. ANTIMICROBIAL TREATMENT OF NOSOCOMIAL GASTROINTESTINAL INFECTIONS*

Discontinuation of antibiotics	
and	
Metronidazole†	500 mg q8h PO
or	
Vancomycin	125–250 mg q6h PO

* Virtually always caused by *Clostridium difficile*.
† Drug of choice.

TABLE 59.7. COMBINATIONS OF ANTIMICROBIAL AGENTS FOR TREATMENT OF NOSOCOMIAL INFECTIONS ASSOCIATED WITH IMPLANTABLE CENTRAL NERVOUS SYSTEM DEVICES

Vancomycin	15–20 mg/kg IV q12h IV
with cefotaxime	2 g q4–6h IV
or	
Vancomycin	2 g q12h IV
with gentamicin	2 mg/kg q8h*

*May result in low cerebrospinal fluid levels.

TABLE 59.8. DRUGS OF CHOICE, ARRANGED BY SPECIFIC ORGANISMS, FOR THE TREATMENT OF INFECTION IN CRITICALLY ILL PATIENTS

Organism	Antimicrobial Agent of Choice	Alternative Agents
Gram-positive cocci (aerobic)		
Staphylococcus aureus		
Non-penicillinase-producing	Penicillin	Vancomycin, cephalosporin
Penicillinase-producing	Nafcillin, oxacillin	Vancomycin, cephalosporin
α-Streptococci (*S. viridans*)	Penicillin	Erythromycin, clindamycin, cephalosporin
β-Streptococci (A, B, C, G)	Penicillin	Cephalosporin, erythromycin
Streptococcus faecalis		
Serious infection	Penicillin or ampicillin and aminoglycoside	Vancomycin and aminoglycoside
Uncomplicated urinary tract infection	Ampicillin	Vancomycin
Streptococcus bovis	Penicillin	Cephalosporin, vancomycin

(*continued*)

TABLE 59.8. CONTINUED

Organism	Antimicrobial Agent of Choice	Alternative Agents
Streptococcus pneumoniae	Penicillin	Erythromycin, vancomycin, cephalosporin
Gram-positive bacilli (aerobic)		
Corynebacterium, group JK	Vancomycin	
Gram-negative bacilli (aerobic)		
Acinetobacter sp.	Imipenem	Penicillin and gentamicin, aminoglycoside, ceftazidime, trimethoprim-sulfamethoxazole
Campylobacter sp.	Erythromycin or quinolone	Tetracycline, gentamicin
Enterobacter sp.	Imipenem	Cefotaxime, ceftriaxone, ceftazidime, aminoglycoside
Haemophilus influenzae	Third- or fourth-generation cephalosporin	Aminoglycoside, extended-spectrum penicillin
Escherichia coli	Third- or fourth-generation cephalosporin	Trimethoprim-sulfamethoxazole
Klebsiella pneumoniae	Third- or fourth-generation cephalosporin	Aminoglycoside, aztreonam, extended-spectrum penicillin

Other *Proteus* sp.	Cefotaxime, ceftriaxone, ceftazidime	Aminoglycoside, aztreonam, imipenem
Providencia sp.	Cefotaxime, ceftriaxone, ceftazidime	Aminoglycoside, imipenem, extended-spectrum penicillin
Pseudomonas aeruginosa	Aminoglycoside and extended-spectrum penicillin	Ceftazidime, aztreonam, imipenem, cefepime
Salmonella sp.	Cefotaxime, ceftriaxone, quinolone	Ampicillin, trimethoprim-sulfamethoxazole
Serratia marcescens	Cefotaxime, ceftriaxone, ceftazidime	Aminoglycoside, imipenem, aztreonam
Shigella sp.	Quinolone	Cefotaxime, ceftriaxone, ceftazidime
Anaerobes		
Anaerobic streptococci	Penicillin	Clindamycin
Bacteroides sp.	Penicillin or clindamycin	Metronidazole
Oropharyngeal strains		

(continued)

TABLE 59.8. CONTINUED

Organism	Antimicrobial Agent of Choice	Alternative Agents
Gastrointestinal strains	Metronidazole	Cefoxitin, clindamycin, imipenem, ticarcillin-clavulanic acid, piperacillin-tazobactam
Clostridium sp. (except *C. difficile*)	Penicillin	Clindamycin, metronidazole, imipenem
Clostridium difficile	Metronidazole	Vancomycin
Other bacteria		
Actinomyces and *Arachnia*	Penicillin G	Tetracycline, clindamycin
Nocardia sp.	Trimethoprim-sulfamethoxazole	Tetracycline, imipenem
Mycobacterium tuberculosis	Isoniazid and rifampin and pyrazinamide and ethambutol	Streptomycin, ciprofloxacin, cycloserine, capreomycin, ethionamide

Modified from Abramowicz M, ed. The choice of antibacterial drugs. *Med Lett Drugs Ther* 1996;38:25–34. With permission of *The Medical Letter*.

Chapter 60

Management of Hematologic Complications and Transfusion

PRACTICAL NOTES

- Anemia may be an indicator of critical illness alone, and blood transfusion is advised when the hemoglobin level is 7–9 g/dL. Transfusion strategy in the NICU is not well defined.
- Thrombocytopenia may be related to heparin use, including IV heparin flushes, or to subcutaneously administered heparin. HIT antibodies can be easily detected by enzyme-linked immunosorbent assay.
- Blood product use is associated with risks varying from minor febrile reaction to fatal lung injury.

TABLE 60.1. CAUSES OF ANEMIA
IN THE NICU

Blood loss	Frequent sampling
	Multitrauma
	Neurosurgical intervention
	Retroperitoneal hematoma
Reduced red blood cell production	Drug-induced sepsis or multiorgan failure
	Adverse drug reaction
	Myelosuppression
	Carbamazepine
	Furosemide
	Indomethacin
	Phenobarbital
	Phenothiazine
	Phenytoin
Hemolysis	Phenobarbital
	Phenytoin
	Cephalosporins
	Erythromycin
	NSAIDs
	Omeprazole
	Ketoconazole

NSAIDs, nonsteroidal anti-inflammatory drugs.

TABLE 60.2. CAUSES OF NEW-ONSET THROMBOCYTOPENIA

Sepsis

Diffuse intravascular coagulation

Massive transfusions (> 50% of blood volume)

Heparin use (unfractionated, low-molecular weight heparin)

Drug use (e.g., rifampin, sulfonamides, vancomycin, carbamazepine, phenytoin, valproic acid, cimetidine, famotidine, acetaminophen, chlorothiazide)

TABLE 60.3. ESTIMATED BLOOD TRANSFUSION RISKS

Transfusion associated related lung injury (1 in 5,000)

Bacterial contamination (1 in 15,000)

Hepatitis B (1 in 130,000)

Severe hemolytic reaction (1 in 600,000)

Hepatitis C (1 in 1,000,000)

Human immunodeficiency virus (1 in 1,200,000)

West Nile virus (minimal)

Chapter 62

Management of Drug Reactions

PRACTICAL NOTES

- Side effects are common but rarely consequential leading to major comorbidity.
- Drug interactions are complicated and rarely sufficiently understood.
- Polypharmacy changes pharmacodynamics in NICU.
- Major skin lesions may include pustulosis and generalized redness.

TABLE 62.1. COMMON DRUG
INTERACTIONS IN THE NICU

Warfarin and Valproic Acid
Mode of action: Drug displacement in protein-
binding site; a high loading dose reaching a higher
serum level may displace warfarin from a valproic
acid binding site.

Phenytoin and Fluconazole
Mode of action: Fluconazole inhibits phenytoin
metabolism and may increase phenytoin level up
to 4 times. Serum concentration monitoring with a
reduction in phenytoin dosage is warranted.

Valproic Acid and Carbapenems
Mode of action: The exact mechanism is unknown.
Carbapenems, especially meropenem, may inhibit
valproic acid absorption. Meropenem may accelerate
the renal excretion and may result in low valproic
acid serum level and increase risk of seizures.
Additionally, carbapenems lower seizure threshold.

Statin and Levofloxacin or Amiodarone
Mode of action: The exact mechanism is unknown,
but severe rhabdomyolysis may occur.

Clopidogrel and Omeprazole
Mode of action: Omeprazole inhibits CYP2C19,
which is responsible for the conversion of clopidogrel
into its active form. The effect of clopidogrel is
reduced up to 47%.

TABLE 62.2. DRUG-INDUCED DERMATOLOGICAL INJURY

Adverse Drug Reaction			Clinical Pharmacology (DoTS)
Reaction	Paradigm Cause	Associated Features	Time from Drug Exposure to Onset
Acute generalized erythematous pustulosis	Diltiazem	Fever > 38°C, neutrophilia, facial edema	Days to weeks (slow time course with diltiazem)
	Erythromycin	Fever > 38°C, neutrophilia, facial edema	Hours to days (rapid time course with antibiotics)
Angioedema due to Type I hypersensitivity	Penicillin	Anaphylactic shock	Minutes
Drug reaction with eosinophilia and systemic symptoms	Phenytoin	Lymphadenopathy, fever, hepatitis, nephritis, pulmonary infiltrates, eosinophilia	Days to weeks
Exanthems	Ampicillin		Days
Fixed drug eruption	Barbiturates		Hours

Phototoxicity	Amiodarone		Months (reaction appears minutes to hours after sun exposure)
Red person syndrome	Vancomycin	Hypotension	Minutes
Scleromyxedema	Gadolinium contrast media	Systemic fibrosis	Many months
Stevens-Johnson syndrome/ toxic epidermal necrolysis	Carbamazepine	Fever, dysphagia, dysuria, conjunctivitis, leukopenia	Days to weeks

DoTS, dose, time-course, susceptibility. Adapted from Ferner RE.[5]

TABLE 62.3. ETIOLOGIES OF EXTRAVASATION BY RISK FACTOR CATEGORY

Category	Risk Factors
Infusion-specific factors	Duration of infusion
	Infiltration volume
	Catheter gauge (relative to vein size)
	Inadequately secured catheter
	Catheter type (steel > Teflon > polyurethane)
	Infusion rate
	Catheter location in elbow, ankle, dorsum of hand, or any other point of flexion
	Multiple venous access attempts proximal to site of venous access
	Need for catheter readjustments

Part XII Decisions at the End of Life and Other Responsibilities

Chapter 63

The Diagnosis of Brain Death

PRACTICAL NOTES

- Brain death can be determined accurately with a neuro-logic examination but only after hypothermia, drug effects, and acute metabolic derangements have been excluded.
- Apnea testing requires an apneic oxygenation method aiming at Pco_2 of 60 mm Hg or an increase of 20 mm Hg above baseline. With an estimated increase of 3–6 mm Hg per minute, 8 minutes is required to reach the target.
- Preoxygenation, increasing temperature to normother-mia, and adequate fluid status reduce complications during apnea testing.
- Diabetes insipidus and hypotension is best treated with infusions of norepinephrine and vasopressin.

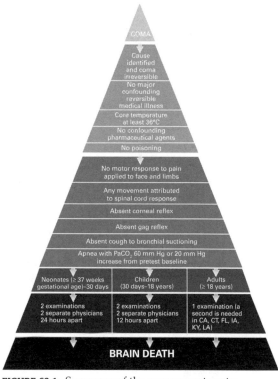

FIGURE 63.1: Summary of the necessary steps to diagnose brain death.

TABLE 63.1. PITFALLS OF
ANCILLARY TESTS

Cerebral angiogram

- Injection aortic arch or individually catheterizing cerebral arteries may make a difference in result. Force of the injection may determine filling or not.
- No guidelines for interpretation

Transcranial Doppler

- Technical difficulties and skill may make a difference in result
- Normal early in anoxic-ischemic brain injury and in primary infratentorial lesions without extreme hydrocephalus

Electroencephalography

- ICU Artifacts
- Measures mostly cortical activity

Somatosensory evoked potentials

- Absent in patients with catastrophic CNS lesions but who are not brain dead

MR angiogram

- Certain techniques or gadolinium use may make a difference in result

CT angiogram

- Interpretation difficulties due to rapid acquisition time
- Retained blood flow in many arterial territories of uncertain significance

Nuclear brain scan

- Areas of perfusion in thalamus in anoxic ischemic brain injury or in patients with a skull defect

Chapter 64

Donation after Cardiac Death

PRACTICAL NOTES

- Donation after cardiac death has been accepted as an alternative procedure for organ donation, mostly for patients who have a catastrophic neurologic disease and as part of the implementation of withdrawal of life support.
- The impact on the donor pool is small, but donation using DCD protocols has gradually increased over the years.
- Better prediction is possible using the DCD-N score. In current DCD data sets, 20% of patients do not proceed to cardiac arrest in the operating suite.

TABLE 64.1. PREREQUISITES
IN DONATION AFTER CARDIAC DEATH
PROTOCOL

Eligibility criteria are satisfied.[a]

All procedures have been explained to the patient's relatives or proxy.

Consent has been given for withdrawal of support (comfort care).

Consent has been given for organ donation.

The appropriateness of the opioids or sedatives for the patients' needs has been determined and discussed with the family.

Family support has been provided.

Death will be determined by a physician with no moral objections to this practice and who is separate from the organ procurement team.

[a] Excluded from the protocol are prior history of intravenous drug use; sepsis or other serious infection; active malignancies; prior infections with human T-cell leukemia-lymphoma virus; systemic viral infection; and prior related disease.

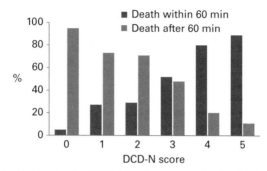

FIGURE 64.2: The DCD-N scale predicts death within 1 hour. Taking into account the presence or absence of corneal reflexes (one point), absent cough reflex (two points), absent motor response or extensor responses (one point), or an increased oxygenation index of > 3 [100 x (FiO_2 x mean airway pressure in cm H_2O/PaO_2 in mm Hg)] (one point). Graph shows probabilities.

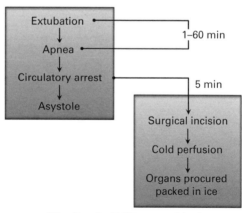

FIGURE 64.3: Timeline for DCD protocol in the operating room.

Chapter 65

Organ Procurement

PRACTICAL NOTES

- Organ donation agencies become involved before brain death declaration but operational only after brain death declaration.
- Most families understand the process of organ donation very well and agree to proceed in 60% to 80% of cases.
- Discussions about organ donation are detailed and the responsibility of organ donation agencies.
- The neurointensivist plays an important coordinating role in the process of organ donation.

Chapter 66

Ethical and Legal Matters

PRACTICAL NOTES

- Do-not-resuscitate orders should be actively discussed.
- Withdrawal of support is a shared decision
- Continuous communication may resolve conflicts
- Adequate documentation, disclosure, and candor should be part of standard care.

PART XIII Formulas and Scales

Formulas and Tables for Titrating Therapy

This appendix provides common formulas and nomograms for calculations needed in the daily care of critically ill neurologic patients. The focus is on patients with an acute neurologic disorder. Standard critical care textbooks and pharmaceutical textbooks in critical care can be consulted as well, and ideally should be available in every neurosciences intensive care unit (NICU). Calculations can also be found on the Internet (www.medcalc.com).

GAS EXCHANGE CALCULATION

$FIO2$ Fraction of inspired oxygen: 0.21– 1.0
PB Barometric pressure at sea level: 760 mm Hg
PH_2O Partial pressure of H_2O: 47 mm Hg (at 37°C)

$$RQ = \frac{VCO_2}{VO_2} = normal = 0.8$$

Calculation for alveolar- arterial (A – a) PO_2 gradient

1. $PAO_2 = FIO_2(PB - PH_2O) - \dfrac{PACO_2}{RQ}$

    $= FIO_2(713) - \dfrac{PAO_2}{0.8}$

2. Measure PO_2 from blood gas
    $PAO_2 - PO_2 = 10 – 20$ mm Hg

WATER DEFICIT

$$\text{Total body water deficit} = 0.6 \times \text{body weight}(\text{kg}) \times \left(\frac{\text{serum Na}}{140 - 1} \right)$$

(assuming 140 mmol/L is desired serum sodium)

OSMOLAL GAP

$$\text{Calculated plasma osmolarity} = 2 \times (\text{Na}) + \frac{(\text{glucose})}{18}$$
$$+ \frac{(\text{blood urea nitrogen}[\text{BUN}])}{2.8}$$
$$= \text{mOsm}/\text{kg}$$

Measured plasma osmolarity = 275–295 mOsm/kg
Osmolar gap = measured Posm– Pcalc = ≤ 10 mOsm/kg

ANION GAP

$$\text{Anion gap} = \text{unmeasured anions} - \text{unmeasured cations}$$
$$= \text{Na}^+ - (\text{Cl}^- + \text{HCO}_3^-)$$
$$= 12 \text{ mEq}/\text{L}$$

ADULT ENTERAL NUTRITION FORMULARY

Formula (Brand)	kcal/mL	Protein (g/L)	Osmolality (mOsm/kg)	Volume to Meet US RDA	Indications for Use
Osmolite HN	1.06	44	300	1,320	Standard formula
Promote	1.0	62.5	340	1,000	Stressed patients with higher protein requirements and intact hepatic and renal function
Osmolite	1.06	37	300	1,887	Patients with lower protein requirements or protein restriction
Peptamen	1.0	40	270 (unflavored) 380 (flavored)	1,500	Patients with severe gastrointestinal disease or pancreatic insufficiency

(continued)

			(CONTINUED)	
Sustacal Plus	1.52	61	670	1,184	Hypercaloric oral supplement
Nutren 1.5	1.5	60	410 (unflavored)	1,000	Hypercaloric tube-feeding formula

RDA, recommended dietary allowance.
Note: Propofol provides 1.1 kcal/mL.

DOSAGE ADJUSTMENT OF ANTIMICROBIAL AGENTS IN RENAL FAILURE*

	Glomerular Filtration Rate (mL/min)		
	> 50	10–50	< 10
Aminoglycosides			
Gentamicin	8–12	12	24
Tobramycin	8–12	12	24
Antifungal agents			
Amphotericin B	24	24	24–36
Flucytosine	6	12–24	24–48
Antiviral agents			
Acyclovir	8	24	48
Amantadine	12–24	48–72	168

(continued)

(CONTINUED)

Cephalosporins			
Cefamandole	6	6–8	8
Cefazolin	6	12	24–48
Cefotaxime	6–8	8–12	12–24
Cefoxitin	8	8–12	24–48
Cephalothin	6	6	8–12
Antibiotics			
Clindamycin	None	None	None
Erythromycin	None	None	None
Metronidazole	8	8–12	12–24
Penicillins			
Amoxicillin	6	6–12	12–16
Ampicillin	6	6–12	12–16
Carbenicillin	8–12	12–24	24–48
Dicloxacillin	None	None	None
Nafcillin	None	None	None
Penicillin G	6–8	8–12	12–16

Piperacillin	4–6	6–8	8
Ticarcillin	8–12	12–24	24–28
Sulfas/trimethoprim			
Sulfamethoxazole	12	18	24
Trimethoprim	12	18	24
Tetracyclines			
Doxycycline	12	12–18	18–24
Minocycline	None	None	None
Vancomycin	12–24	72–240	240

* Interval extension in hours.

Modified from Bennett WM, Arnoff GR, Golper TA, et al. *Drug Prescribing in Renal Failure.* Philadelphia: American College of Physicians; 1987. With permission of the publisher.

DRUGS THAT ALTER ANTIEPILEPTIC DRUG (AED) CONCENTRATIONS

Mechanism of Drug Interaction	Carbamazepine	Phenobarbital	Phenytoin	Valproic Acid
Changes in AED absorption				
Protein-binding displacement			Antacids Enteral feedings Salicylates Sulfas Valproic acid	Salicylates
Enzyme inhibition of AED	Cimetidine Danazol Diltiazem Erythromycin Fluoxetine Isoniazid Propoxyphene Valproic acid Verapamil	Chloramphenicol Cimetidine Isoniazid Valproic acid	Amiodarone Chloramphenicol Cimetidine Ciprofloxacin Disulfiram Isoniazid Omeprazole Phenylbutazone Propoxyphene	

Enzyme induction of AED	Phenobarbital Phenytoin Primidone	Carbamazepine Ethanol Phenytoin	Carbamazepine Ethanol Phenobarbital	Carbamazepine Phenobarbital Primidone Phenytoin
Enzyme induction of AED on other drugs	Clonazepam Doxycycline Ethosuximide Theophylline Valproic acid Warfarin	Carbamazepine Chlorpromazine Corticosteroids Doxycycline Oral contraceptives Phenytoin Quinidine Tricyclic antidepressants Warfarin	Carbamazepine Corticosteroids Doxycycline Folic acid Oral contraceptives Primidone Pyridoxine Quinidine Vitamin D Warfarin	
Enzyme inhibition				Ethosuximide Phenobarbital Phenytoin Primidone

MODIFIED NATIONAL INSTITUTES OF HEALTH STROKE SCALE*

Item Number	Item Name	Score
1A	Level of consciousness	0 = alert; responsive 1 = not alert; verbally arousable 2 = not alert; only responsive to repeated stimuli 3 = totally unresponsive
1B	Level of consciousness questions	0 = answers both correctly 1 = answers one correctly 2 = answers neither correctly
1C	Level of consciousness commands	0 = performs both tasks correctly 1 = performs one task correctly 2 = performs neither task
2	Gaze	0 = normal 1 = partial gaze palsy 2 = forced gaze deviation

3	Visual fields	0 = no visual loss
		1 = partial hemianopsia
		2 = complete hemianopsia
5a	Left arm	0 = no drift
		1 = drift before 10 seconds
		2 = falls before 10 seconds
		3 = no effort against gravity
		4 = no movement
5b	Right arm	0 = no drift
		1 = drift before 10 seconds
		2 = falls before 10 seconds
		3 = no effort against gravity
		4 = no movement
6a	Left leg	0 = no drift
		1 = drift before 5 seconds
		2 = falls before 5 seconds
		3 = no effort against gravity
		4 = no movement

(continued)

(CONTINUED)

6b	Right leg	0 = no drift
		1 = drift before 5 seconds
		2 = falls before 5 seconds
		3 = no effort against gravity
		4 = no movement
8	Sensory	0 = normal
		1 = abnormal
9	Language	0 = normal
		1 = mild aphasia
		2 = severe aphasia
		3 = mute or global aphasia
11	Neglect	0 = normal
		1 = mild
		2 = severe

*The item numbers correspond to the numbering in the original scale to allow easy identification of the changes. From Lyden PD, Lu M, Levine SR, et al. A modified National Institutes of Health Stroke Scale for use in stroke clinical trials: preliminary reliability and validity. *Stroke* 2001;32:1310–1317. With permission of the American Heart Association.

TABLE 8.2 DETERMINING THE INTRACRANIAL HEMORRHAGE (ICH) SCORE

Component	ICH Score Points
Glasgow Coma Scale (GCS)	
3–4	2
5–12	1
13–15	0
ICH volume (mL)	
> 30	1
< 30	0
Intraventricular hemorrhage (IVH)	
Yes	1
No	0
Infratentorial origin of ICH	
Yes	1
No	0
Age (years)	
> 80	1
< 80	0
Total ICH score	0-6

ICH, intracerebral hemorrhage; GCS = GCS score on initial presentation (or after resuscitation).
ICH volume on initial CT calculated using ABC12 method.
IVH indicates presence of any intraventricular hemorrhage on initial computed tomography.
From Hemphill JC, 3rd, Bonovich DC, Besmertis L, Manley GT, Johnston SC. The ICH score: a simple, reliable grading scale for intracerebral hemorrhage. *Stroke* 2001;32:891–897.

STANDARD NEUROLOGICAL CLASSIFICATION OF SPINAL CORD INJURY

MOTOR
KEY MUSCLES

	R	L	
C2			
C3			
C4			
C5			Elbow flexors
C6			Wrist extensors
C7			Elbow extensors
C8			Finger flexors (distal phalanx of middle finger)
T1			Finger abductors (little finger)

0 = total paralysis
1 = palpable or visible contraction
2 = active movement,
    gravity eliminated
3 = active movement,
    against gravity
4 = active movement,
    against some resistance
5 = active movement,
    against full resistance
NT = not testable

	R	L	
L2			Hip flexors
L3			Knee extensors
L4			Ankle dorsiflexors
L5			Long toe extensors
S1			Ankle plantar flexors

☐ Voluntary anal contraction (Yes/No)

TOTALS ☐ + ☐ = ☐ MOTOR SCORE
(MAXIMUM) (50) (50) (100)

SENSORY
KEY SENSORY POINTS

	LIGHT TOUCH		PIN PRICK	
	R	L	R	L
C2				
C3				
C4				
C5				
C6				
C7				
C8				
T1				
T2				
T3				
T4				
T5				
T6				
T7				
T8				
T9				
T10				
T11				
T12				
L1				
L2				
L3				
L4				
L5				
S1				
S2				
S3				
S4-5				

0 = absent
1 = impaired
2 = normal
NT = not testable

'Key Sensory Points

☐ Any anal sensation (Yes/No)

TOTALS { ☐ ☐ = ☐ PIN PRICK SCORE (max. 112)
(MAXIMUM) (56) (56) (56) (50)
        ☐ ☐ = ☐ LIGHT TOUCH SCORE (max. 112)

NEUROLOGICAL LEVEL
The most caudal segment with normal function

	R	L
SENSORY	☐	☐
MOTOR	☐	☐

COMPLETE OR INCOMPLETE? ☐
Incomplete = Any sensory or motor function in S4-S5

ASIA IMPAIRMENT SCALE ☐

ZONE OF PARTIAL PRESERVATION
Caudal extent of partially innervated segments

	R	L
SENSORY	☐	☐
MOTOR	☐	☐

2000 Rev.

This form may be copied freely but should not be altered without permission from the American Spinal Injury Association.